Strength Training for *W*omen

James A. Peterson, PhD, FACSM
StairMaster Sports/Medical Products, Inc.
Kirkland, WA

Cedric X. Bryant, PhD, FACSM
StairMaster Sports/Medical Products, Inc.
Kirkland, WA

Susan L. Peterson, MS
Microsoft Corporation
Redmond, WA

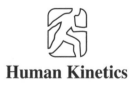

Human Kinetics

Library of Congress Cataloging-in-Publication Data

Peterson, James A., 1943-
    Strength training for women / James A. Peterson, Cedric X. Bryant,
Susan L. Peterson.
        p. cm.
    Includes index.
    ISBN: 0-87322-752-2 (pbk.)
    1. Weight training for women.   2. Physical education and training.
3. Muscle strength. I. Bryant, Cedric X., 1960- . II. Peterson,
Susan L.   III. Title.
GV546.6.W64P47   1995
613.7'13--dc20   94-47646
                                                                 CIP

ISBN: 0-87322-752-2

Developmental Editors: Mary E. Fowler, Anne M. Heiles; **Assistant Editors:** Ed Giles, Karen Grieves, Dawn Roselund, Henry Woolsey, and Rebecca Ewert; **Copyeditor:** Denelle Eknes; **Proofreader:** Anne Meyer Byler; **Indexer:** Barbara E. Cohen; **Typesetting and Layout:** Ruby Zimmerman; **Text Design and Layout:** Stuart Cartwright; **Cover Design:** Jody Boles; **Photographer (cover):** Chris Brown; **Photographer (interior):** Gordon Modine and Deborah de Maio; **Cover Model:** Vilia Bailey; **Interior Models:** Mary Adams, Lisa Johnson, Ginger Bryant, Carol Herlihy, Mary Lynn Laker, Tiffany Mason, B.J. Powell, Carol Lorenz, and Jessica Eller; **Printer:** Versa Press

Human Kinetics books are available at special discounts for bulk purchase. Special editions or book excerpts can also be created to specification. For details, contact the Special Sales Manager at Human Kinetics.

Printed in the United States of America   10 9 8 7 6 5 4 3 2

Human Kinetics
P.O. Box 5076, Champaign, IL 61825-5076
1-800-747-4457

Canada: Human Kinetics, Box 24040, Windsor, ON N8Y 4Y9
1-800-465-7301 (in Canada only)

Europe: Human Kinetics, P.O. Box IW14, Leeds LS16 6TR, United Kingdom
(44) 1132 781708

Australia: Human Kinetics, 2 Ingrid Street, Clapham 5062, South Australia
(08) 371 3755

New Zealand: Human Kinetics, P.O. Box 105-231, Auckland 1
(09) 523 3462

Contents

Foreword

During my lifetime, I have constantly been reminded of the importance of a woman's level of muscular fitness and its effect on the quality of her life. As a five-time member of the United States Olympic team, I have seen the enormous impact of a high level of muscular fitness, not only in the remarkable achievements of my Olympic teammates, but also in the ability of strength to prevent injuries in physically active people.

As a health care professional, I have also had the opportunity to observe how muscular fitness can affect the ability of individuals to perform the basic tasks of daily living. Without question, an adequate level of strength is an essential component of a healthy lifestyle. From carrying groceries to climbing stairs, whether you work at a desk or on your feet, muscular fitness will enable you to better handle the physical demands and challenges inherent in your lifestyle.

Strength Training for Women offers women of all ages and fitness levels a user-friendly guide on developing muscular fitness. The book provides an overview of the importance of strength training on a regular basis and a much-needed summary of the parameters of sensible, medically sound strength training.

Strength Training for Women was written to help you—whether you're just starting a strength training program or want to improve an existing training regimen. I particularly enjoyed the chapters that explain why and how women should conquer their inhibitions regarding strength training and on strength training without equipment. The authors do an excellent job of dispelling much of the misinformation which is associated with strength training. In addition, they explain clearly why cost should not be a prohibitive factor in designing a safe, effective strength training program.

Aptly and abundantly illustrated, this book is must reading for any woman who wants to take care of her most important asset—her health. As a woman, a key question you should ask yourself is: "Should I make strength training an integral part of my exercise regimen?" Of course, you should. In countless ways, the quality of your life depends on it. The authors of *Strength Training for Women* have shown you the way. The next step is yours. The authors have provided a powerful recipe of "real exercise for real people." Their recipe can help you enhance the quality of your life. Bon appetit!

Willye White
Former Olympic track and field athlete

Preface

Virtually everyone—young or old, male or female—can experience improvements in muscular fitness. If you want to have stronger, more durable muscles and bones, improve your physical appearance, and enhance your self-image, then strength training is for you. By committing yourself to a strength training program, you've taken the first step in improving your muscle strength and endurance (muscular fitness). You have affirmed the fact that you understand and appreciate the importance of muscular fitness and sensible training.

Any attempt you make to increase your level of muscular fitness may be somewhat unproductive, however, if you do not adhere to proper techniques and training principles. Over the years we've discovered that sensible training methods combined with desire and effort result in optimal improvements in muscular fitness. One without the other is an unwise and ineffective compromise.

During the past two decades we've had the opportunity to advise and train many women on enhancing their physical fitness and overall wellness. These women represent diverse backgrounds and interests and have come from all walks of life—the United States Military Academy at West Point, Pepsi Cola Worldwide, Microsoft, the Avon Women's Running Program, and various elements of the American public school system—to name a few. Some women were older than others. Some were more fit. Some were more motivated to exercise. Some worked with their hands, while others had more administrative and clerical occupations. But each, in her own way, contributed to our understanding and belief that a sound strength training program can enhance the quality of life for women of all ages. That belief is the fundamental premise for *Strength Training for Women.*

We wrote this book to give easy-to-understand, easy-to-follow instructions to women on developing muscular fitness. Although the situation appears to be improving, we have found that many women have a relatively limited understanding of the topic. Of those women who do regularly spend time strength training, many engage in efforts that are woefully incapable of achieving the intended objectives. We want to change that. The readable information we present will let you develop a personalized program to meet your personal goals whether you have never lifted a weight before or you are an experienced lifter.

Strength Training for Women features techniques and programs designed to be appropriate for a variety of training interests. For example, we present specific programs for 13 different sports. There's also a section on how to strength train without using equipment. We explain buddy exercises and negative-only exercises (based primarily on efforts undertaken at West Point to accommodate new cadets, who often arrive as plebes with insufficient levels of upper body muscular fitness) and their extraordinary ability to develop strength both quickly and safely. Other special features include a listing of sample strength training programs and a chapter on how you can firm up your body.

This book is divided into three parts. The first explains why muscle strength and endurance are important. Chapter 1 presents the benefits of strength training and dispels several common myths and misconceptions about strength training. It also looks at special issues—nutrition, common questions, age, and prenatal and postnatal training. Chapter 2 shows you how to organize your strength training program to maximize results safely and efficiently. In chapter 3 we provide information on all types of strength training equipment, and help you decide what's best for you. We also share tips for selecting a workout environment that will best meet your needs.

An illustrated guide on how to perform basic strength training exercises appears in Part II. Properly performed, each exercise offers you a tested way of developing strength safely, effectively, and efficiently. Most of these exercises are used at the United States Military Academy—arguably an institution with the most physically fit student body in the world. The chapters in this section focus on exercises that can be done with a particular type of equipment (free weights, multistation equipment, variable resistance machines) or approach (strength training without weights).

The third part of the book presents strength training guidelines and advice for specific groups or exercise interests. Chapter 8 outlines sample workouts for the most commonly used programs of strength training. Chapter 9 discusses how and why athletes should strength train. Chapter 10 explains what you can do if you want to firm up your body.

More and more women have accepted that strength training is an essential component of any functional conditioning program. By better preparing individuals to handle the demands of daily living—both at work and at play—higher levels of muscular fitness can have a critical impact on quality of life. With *Strength Training for Women*, you have an easy-to-use blueprint for achieving the level of muscular fitness you need and deserve. Let's get started.

Dedication

To our nine nieces—Eileen, Jamie, Krista, Ledia, Michelle, Rachel, Rebecca, Samantha, and Susie. May they live in a world that realizes that "muscles do matter" for women of all ages.

Acknowledgments

The authors are grateful to the many individuals at Human Kinetics who provided professional assistance of the highest level—particularly Rainer Martens, the publisher. We would also like to express our appreciation to Roseanne Kiesz for her invaluable typing assistance.

PART

I

GETTING STARTED

So, you've decided to strength train. You've made a good choice. Although you recognize the value of strength training, it can seem very complicated. In the first three chapters, we'll clear up the confusion and myths surrounding strength training and give you the facts—facts that will help you set your goals, design a program to meet those goals, and put you into the best position to enjoy the benefits of your efforts.

We begin chapter 1 by outlining the benefits of strength training and describing how it has worked for women of all ages and lifestyles. Some benefits you might already know; others may be new to you. You'll find this information helpful if you want to improve your performance (not just in sporting activities, but in everyday life), enrich your physical health, uplift your mental health, and enhance your appearance. We'll help you conquer your fears about strength training and dispel the 15 most common myths that cloud women's views of the activity.

Based on this information, we'll help you set realistic goals for your strength training program and lead you through the steps to develop a strength training plan. Most women want their strength training program to

- produce the optimum results,
- require a minimum of time, and
- place a premium on their personal safety.

We also look at some issues that are specific to women who want to strength train. Nutrition is an important part of any exercise program and especially important for women. We have included a discussion of nutrition to clarify the changes you might need to make in your eating habits when involved in a strength training program. We'll also dispel the myths behind some popular food and vitamin supplements that are better for making their producers money than they are for your physical health. As the chapter continues you'll find guidelines for women who face specific issues—seniors, adolescents, and pregnant and postpartum women. Sprinkled throughout the chapter are common questions that women have about the effects of strength training on their lives and bodies.

Chapter 2 will help you achieve the goals you've identified. We talk about ways to design your plan to stay focused and motivated. We show you how to assess your strength from the beginning so that you won't become discouraged by jumping in too hard, too soon. We'll also teach you the basics of strength training to familiarize you with terms that you'll hear in the weight room. And we'll instruct you on techniques that will minimize your chances for injury while maximizing your chances for success.

Once you've designed your program and have

a strength training plan, you need to select your equipment and decide where to do your training. In chapter 3, we present and outline the advantages and disadvantages of the most commonly used equipment—free weights, multistation machines, and variable resistance machines. We even give you tips to achieve high results using low-cost equipment such as resistance cords and sticks.

You've seen the positive results strength training has on others, but you also know women who have failed in their strength training efforts. The chapters in Part I will give you information to lessen your chances for failure. Let's get you started on your road to success.

CHAPTER 1

FEELING STRONG ABOUT GETTING FIT

Everyone has different reasons for committing to a strength training program. Some women want to improve their abilities to perform specific tasks, others want to improve their physical and mental health, and still others simply desire a more toned and shapely appearance. Whatever your goals, sticking with a strength training program based on medically sound guidelines will put you well on your way. And it won't take long to begin seeing results.

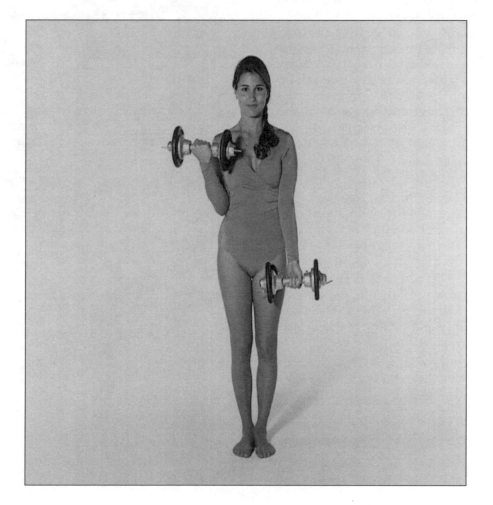

THE BENEFITS OF STRENGTH TRAINING

The benefits of strength training are numerous. Simply stated, strength training can meet the needs and interests of a wide variety of people. Let's take a look at what it's doing for Ginger, Mary, and Lisa.

Ginger, aged 27, began lifting weights to improve her strength after giving birth to her second child. She had noticed that her back and upper body were frequently sore as she carried her children, their car seats, and endless other items from place to place. Time to exercise was limited now that Ginger was caring for two children and gearing up a freelance business, but she discovered that she could increase her strength and stamina by training in her home 30 min a day, three times a week. And she doesn't use fancy equipment or a personal trainer—her cost has been surprisingly low.

Mary, who is 65 years old, recently retired and enjoys community service activities. She knows it is important to keep active and, now that her children are grown, doesn't want to become a "tired old grandmother." Mary joined a fitness club, where she lifts weights three mornings a week. In the process, she has met a group of friends with whom she shares other interests. Mary finds herself full of energy and ready to actively enjoy her retirement. She has even toned up her muscles; she looks and feels terrific.

As a former college athlete, **Lisa,** aged 35, is well aware of the benefits of strength training. But she hasn't done much of it since college. Now her body doesn't respond to exercise the way it used to. Lisa wants to play recreational sports, but she is concerned about possible injury. She recently consulted a local fitness expert, and together they developed a strength training program that will help keep Lisa fit for play.

You may see a little of yourself in one or maybe all of these women. Strength training works for them and it can work for you. Let's explore the primary benefits.

IMPROVING YOUR PERFORMANCE

The performance-enhancing aspect of strength training is affected tremendously by your own needs and interests. For example, if you play sports at any competitive level, you are likely to recognize the positive effects of greater muscular fitness on a variety of sport-related skills. But the functional benefits of strength training are not confined to athletes and would-be competitors. Improved muscle strength can make lifting or carrying heavy materials on the job or at home less strenuous. You'll be able to complete such tasks repeatedly with better muscle endurance. And strength training can play a central role in enabling women of all ages to maintain physically active and relatively challenging lifestyles.

One of the cornerstones of independent living is maintaining enough muscular fitness that you can perform your daily tasks—from lifting grocery bags to climbing stairs. The medical community has been excited about recent research demonstrating that proper strength training is invaluable in helping senior citizens maintain independence and personal dignity.

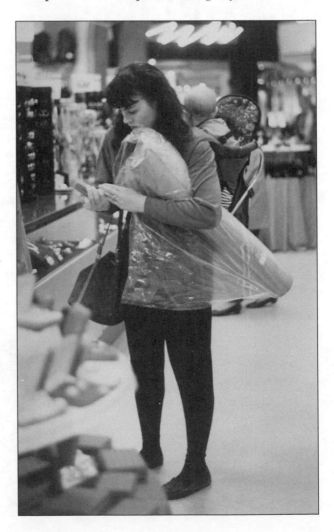

ENRICHING YOUR PHYSICAL HEALTH

A higher level of muscular fitness can greatly reduce your chances of suffering both muscle and skeletal injuries. It's estimated that about half of the various injuries that occur in physical activity could be prevented through greater muscular fitness. So you can view strength training as an effective (and relatively inexpensive) form of health insurance.

Strength training has been found to serve additional health-related roles. Cardiac rehabilitation specialists frequently include strength training exercise (in doses of moderate intensity) to improve the upper body strength of cardiac patients whose muscles have lost tone and function due to physical inactivity. And for people with osteoarthritic conditions, a higher level of fitness in the muscles surrounding the skeletal joints reduces the relative stress the joints must handle and provides some pain relief. Strength training performed over an extended period also increases bone density, which helps to lower your risk of

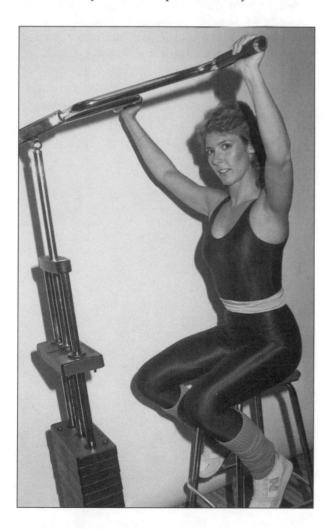

osteoporosis. And strength training seems to play an important role in treating and preventing lower back pain.

UPLIFTING YOUR MENTAL HEALTH

There's no question that having a higher level of muscular fitness will improve how you feel about yourself. As your self-esteem rises, your outlook on other factors in your life tends to improve, too. Research indicates that regular strength training exercise can help you better control and manage stress. Strength training also has been found to improve both the quality and the quantity of sleep. Whether that effect is a by-product of physiological or psychological factors (or both) is relative to your individual circumstances.

ENHANCING YOUR APPEARANCE

Unlike other types of exercise, strength training provides the exerciser with readily apparent feedback. Large changes in the strength and tone of a muscle can occur over a short time. The fit, healthy look is a matter of muscle tone, and muscle tone is a by-product of proper strength training.

CONQUERING YOUR INHIBITIONS

An argument could be made that any woman who considers the positive results of strength training will decide to do this type of exercise. However, many women are unaware of the possible benefits of strength training exercise. Sometimes they are confronted by attitudes that compromise their interest in strength training. These are some common reasons women give for not strength training:

- I've never lifted before; it's too late to start now.
- Aerobic exercise is all I need to be fit.
- It'd be too much of a hassle to learn the proper techniques, and if I didn't, I'd probably get hurt.
- I can't afford it.
- Strength training is for athletes and I don't play sports.
- I'm too busy.
- I have no desire to look like those bodybuilders on television.

Your view of muscular fitness could be clouded by the misconceptions surrounding strength training. Let's refute the 15 most common myths women hear about strength training.

Myth 1: Women can't get strong.
Women can and should develop muscular fitness. Women have a potential for muscular fitness—particularly in their upper bodies—that usually remains untapped. In fact, the "average woman" gains strength at a slightly faster rate than the "average man."

Myth 2: Strength training defeminizes women.
The potential functional, health, mental, and physical benefits of strength training cannot be confined to members of the male domain. Proper strength training—by helping you increase your physical working capacity, improve your body composition, and lower your risk of injury—will make you look and feel better. Tight, firm muscles have nothing to do with the objectionable and patronizing term, defeminizing.

Myth 3: Lifting weights causes bulky muscles.
Women don't have the genetic potential to develop large muscles because they don't have enough of the hormone, testosterone, needed for the development of muscle bulk. While steroids and other artificial means may cause you to bulk up, lifting weights will not.

Myth 4: Strength training makes you muscle-bound.
Muscle-bound is a term that connotes a lack of flexibility. However, proper strength training doesn't make you less flexible; it makes you more flexible. If you keep your muscles loose and supple by regularly going through a full range of motion (a practice of proper strength training), you will stay flexible.

Myth 5: More is better.
With any form of exercise you eventually reach a point of either diminishing or no returns. You take a chance of injuring yourself if you don't use common sense to decide "how much is enough." The quality of your strength training is much more important than the quantity of time you spend. A quality workout of 30 minutes can effectively and safely develop muscular fitness.

Myth 6: No pain, no gain.
A sensible strength training program might be uncomfortable, but should not be painful. It should put a reasonable demand on your muscle systems to increase your strength, without exposing you to an unreasonable risk of injury.

Myth 7: Muscles turn to fat when you stop training.
Muscles cannot turn into fat. They don't have the physiological ability to change from one type of tissue to another. Muscles do have the property of "use it or lose it." If you don't use a muscle, it will literally waste (atrophy) away. When someone has a cast removed from a leg that had been broken, the unused leg muscles look smaller than they were before the injury. If muscle turned to fat, you would see a "fat ball" when the cast was removed, not atrophied leg muscles.

Myth 8: You must take protein supplements to get a fit physique.
Muscular fitness is not enhanced by using protein supplements because your body can't store extra protein. Excess protein is not used to build muscle tissue. It is converted to fat and stored. So if you consume extra protein in addition to your regular diet, any weight gain will probably be fat. Excess protein also can lead to dehydration and loss of urinary calcium. Chronic calcium loss from too much protein increases the risk of osteoporosis, especially in women.

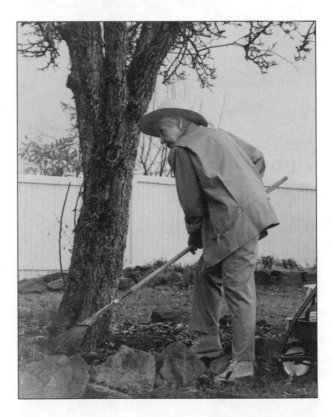

Myth 9: Proper strength training must be complex.

The simpler your approach to strength training, the more likely your efforts will be successful. It can be detrimental to make your strength training program too technical. It can be confusing and can compromise your strength training efforts or can increase the possibility that you won't stick with your training program. Basic muscular development programs—those emphasizing effectiveness, efficiency, and safety over complexity—usually produce the best results.

Myth 10: Proper strength training is expensive.

Muscles respond to the stress applied to them, not to the cost of the machine you train on or the money you spend to join a health and fitness club. Other factors being equal, muscles can't discern 50 lbs of stress on an inexpensive barbell from 50 lbs of stress on a high-tech machine costing thousands of dollars. Your strength training program doesn't even have to involve equipment to be effective, as you will see in chapter 7.

Myth 11: Strength training is a contest.

Individuals who focus on competition in strength training tend to injure themselves or get discouraged and drop out of their programs. It is unrealistic to compare your training numbers (particularly the amount lifted on a specific exercise) with those of other participants. How much you can lift is a by-product of several factors, most of which you have no control over (e.g., the length of your arms or legs). As trite as it may sound, the adage, "do your best and leave the rest," should govern your efforts to develop muscular fitness.

Myth 12: Strength training is for young people.

It's never too late to improve the quality of your life by enjoying a higher level of muscular fitness. Muscular fitness can extend your functional life span. Women in their 90s have improved their levels of muscular fitness and their quality of life by participating in strength training programs.

Myth 13: You'll have a greater need for vitamins.

The vitamin needs of an active person are generally no greater than those of a sedentary one. Vitamins do not contribute significantly to your body structure and do not provide you with a direct source of body energy, so physically active people receive no benefit from taking excessive vitamin supplements. If you eat a variety of healthful foods (breads, cereals, grains, fruits, vegetables, lean meats, etc.), your intake of vitamins will be adequate.

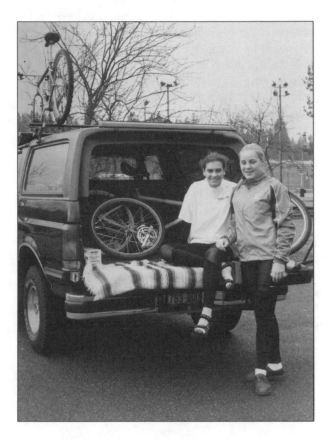

Myth 14: Rigorous strength training rids the body of fat.

Research shows that while strength training can firm and tone muscles, it does not burn away fat. Some fat is needed for normal bodily functions, such as activity in the brain, nerve tissue, heart, bone marrow, and cell membranes. Adult women have about 12% of their body weight in essential fat. For health reasons, the optimal level of total body fat for women should range from 15% to 22%.

Myth 15: Strength training can't be fun.

Strength training can and should be enjoyable. You can design a strength training program that meets your physical needs while being fun. Remember, staying with your exercises is more likely when you enjoy what you're doing.

Some women deal with their inhibitions toward strength training more easily than others. The best approach is learning as much about it as possible. The more informed you are about the effects strength training will have on you, the more you will feel that it is worth the effort.

IDENTIFYING WHICH GOALS ARE RIGHT FOR YOU

Before you begin strength training regularly, take stock of your personal needs. Ask yourself, "Why do I want to strength train?" The answer can help you decide how to train and what program to follow. You may want to strengthen your body for a specific sport (see chapter 9), or supplement a weight-loss program by using strength training to firm up (see chapter 10). We recommend that one of your primary goals should be to handle your body weight when doing push-ups, chin-ups, and dips. Being able to handle your body weight shows that you can use your muscles functionally. The life-enhancing applications of doing a 200-lb bench press are limited. Performing several full-body dips, on the other hand, is a good indicator that you have a high level of torso (upper body) muscular fitness—a quality that affects how well you can use the musculature of your upper body in activities of daily living (lifting a child, moving a piece of furniture, or swinging a golf club).

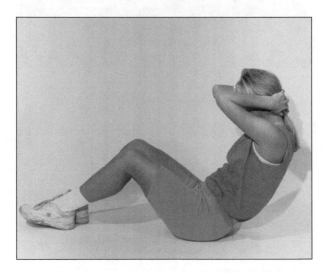

Although you may focus on one objective (such as preventing injuries, increasing performance skills, improving your mental and physical health, improving your appearance, or enhancing the quality of your life), you might notice some additional benefits. For example, getting stronger will not only improve your performance abilities, but also make you less likely to be injured.

Now that you've decided what you want from your strength training program, let's look at how to begin.

ADDRESSING SPECIFIC ISSUES

All women notice changes in their bodies when they begin an exercise program. This chapter deals with common questions women have about these changes and offers suggestions about how to adjust to them or to enjoy them. We'll discuss important nutritional aspects along with the benefits and special considerations you should make if you're a young woman, an older woman, pregnant, or postpartum.

Common Considerations

One of the most frequent questions women have about their bodies during weight training is: What is the effect on my menstrual cycle? Many women have found exercise to help in relieving menstrual discomfort, and there is no evidence that supports ceasing strength training during your menstrual cycle. A good workout can relieve premenstrual tension and alleviate feelings of frustration and irritability. Any discomfort—cramps, heavy or light bleeding—should be shared with your doctor. Sometimes simple prescriptions can put you back on track.

Some women have noticed an irregularity in their menstrual cycles (oligomenorrhea) or even a disappearance of the cycle (amenorrhea). No one knows the cause or the long-term effects of either of these conditions. Some attribute these problems to changes in body fat ratios. Others believe that the stress of training can lead to these conditions. No matter what the cause, it is wise to consult with your doctor or gynecologist if you experience any changes in your menstrual cycle.

ENSURING PROPER NUTRITION

Nutrition can play a substantial role in every aspect of your life. Good nutrition, which involves giving your body specific amounts of essential nutrients, can have a profound impact on your ability to do physical activity, particularly strength training. Essential nutrients can be divided into two main categories—those that provide calories (carbohydrates, protein, and fat) and those that don't provide calories (water, vitamins, and minerals). Nutrients that provide calories supply you with the energy you need to do any physical activity. The noncaloric nutrients don't directly provide energy, but they play a critical role in the biochemical reactions responsible for the energy production.

Proper nutrition is an important component of a sound strength training program. Although no single food or nutrient will turn you into an Olympic champion, poor nutritional habits can prevent you from reaching your genetic potential. Given the significance that nutrition has for physical performance, what should be included in a sound training diet?

Carbohydrates.

Because the major energy source for muscle contraction is from carbohydrates stored in your liver as glycogen, your diet should be high in carbohydrates. A diet that is 55% to 60% carbohydrates will generally maintain your glycogen stores. If you don't eat enough carbohydrates, however, your glycogen stores will eventually become too low. If you eat a diet low in carbohydrates for several days and do intense workouts on those days, your muscle glycogen levels can fall to less than 50% of normal. Such low levels can contribute to feelings of tiredness, soreness, and fatigue. If you had to depend solely on your glycogen stores to support your daily activities, you would run out of energy in less than 24 hours.

Not only should you ensure that your diet is high in carbohydrates, you should also pay attention to the sources of your carbohydrates. Complex carbohydrates or starchy foods (such as pasta, bread, muffins, bagels, rice, potatoes, and cereals), rather than foods high in simple sugar, should make up most of your carbohydrate intake. Although sweets and sugar-laden foods such as soda pop, candy, and desserts can contribute to your glycogen stores, they don't contain essential vitamins and minerals. As a result, if you are a physically active woman, you should eat nutritional, starchy foods, rather than sweets, to build your levels of glycogen.

Protein.

Unfortunately, most physically active women overestimate how much protein they should eat. It is not unusual to find that many physically active women eat at least twice as much protein as they need. The hazards of eating excessive protein over a long time are not clear. However, eating too much protein is believed to have some risks. First, any protein you eat that your body doesn't need isn't stored as protein. Depending on the energy needs of your body, extra protein is either stored as fat or used for energy. To use dietary protein as a source of energy is a very inefficient metabolic process. Dietary carbohydrate is a much better source of energy. Second, when extra dietary protein is metabolized, the nitrogen portion of the protein must be excreted in your urine as urea. To excrete large amounts of urea, water, which must also be excreted, is needed. Research has shown that a diet high in protein increases your risk of dehydration.

As a guideline, nutritional scientists recommend that about 15% of your daily calories come from the protein in foods. Most people find this recommended level surprisingly low. Since physically active women require more protein than inactive women and adolescents require more protein than adults, both groups tend to eat more food. Their higher caloric diets are usually more than adequate to meet their protein needs.

As a strength training enthusiast, you will probably see many advertisements that promote "protein drinks" or "protein powders" for optimal muscle mass development. These so-called developmental products typically contain a carbohydrate and a protein source—both of which do nothing more than add extra calories to your diet. Although optimal muscle development won't happen without enough calories, if you are a typical individual you eat more than enough protein and calories for sound muscle growth. If you buy one of these often expensive "growth" products in the futile hope of enhancing your muscular fitness and size, you are wasting your money. Your efforts would be much better devoted to simply eating a "normal" diet.

Amino Acids.

A newer addition to the marketplace is single amino acid supplements. Amino acids are known as the "building blocks" of proteins because all proteins are made of several amino acids. Eight of these building blocks are considered "essential" because they can't be made or synthesized by your body and, as a result, must be eaten. Healthy, physically active people who eat a normal diet have no need for amino acid supplements. For example, one egg, one 8-oz carton of milk, and 3 oz of tuna fish provide all the essential amino acids that a 130-lb young woman needs. On the other hand, overeating amino acids can have negative consequences. Similar to excess protein, any amino acids you eat that you don't need won't be stored in your body, but will either be inefficiently used or converted to and stored as fat. Amino acid supplementation can also increase your risk of dehydration. These supplements tend to be very expensive and very wasteful.

Fat.

The final nutrient in your training diet that provides calories is fat. As might be expected, the recommended guideline for fat consumption for most people is much lower than what is usually eaten. Many active people get 40% of their calories from fat, although a diet with a fat content of 30% or less is recommended. Unfortunately, calories from fat are often not obvious. For example, one teaspoon of margarine, butter, oil, or mayonnaise contains 45 calories and is pure fat. Not surprisingly, it is easy to eat more fat than you would expect. Because foods that are high in complex carbohydrates or starches are not high in fat, your fat intake normally decreases as you eat more carbohydrates.

Vitamins and Minerals.

The misunderstanding about what constitutes a proper training diet also extends to nutrients that don't have calories. For example, many physically active people believe that they should take vitamin and mineral supplements, because they incorrectly assume that exercise increases their need for vitamins and minerals. Vitamins tend to be recycled and reused, as opposed to used up. Usually, the more you exercise, the more food you eat, and, as a result, the more vitamins and minerals you consume. Women doing strenuous activities such as strength training tend to get more than enough vitamins and minerals through their diets, provided they are consuming at least 1500 calories per day. Research does not support the idea that vitamin and mineral supplementation has a positive effect on physical performance. Megadosing on vitamins (especially A, D, E, and K) and minerals can be potentially harmful to your liver.

Fluids.

Fluids also play an important role in your training diet. Ingesting enough fluid can be critical. Excessive water loss through perspiration can lead to a potentially dangerous situation. A loss of just 3% of your body weight can impair performance. Heat exhaustion can begin when 5% of your body's weight has been lost. To avoid

these conditions, you should drink liberal amounts of water before, during, and after your strength workouts. Each pound of body weight lost during your workout should be replaced with at least 2 cups of water.

The best fluid replacer for a physically active person is cool water. Fluids that contain sugar aren't emptied from the stomach or intestinal tract as quickly as water. If you believe that you need a sugared beverage, diluting a commercial sports drink with 3 parts of water to 1 part beverage is a good compromise.

Sample Menus.

The following menus are examples of high-carbohydrate/low-fat meals that will provide you with about 1500 calories per day.

BREAKFAST OPTIONS

Each of these breakfasts provides about 350 calories from the following food groups: 2 starch servings, 1 fruit serving, 1 milk serving, 1 fat serving (allow 1 egg twice a week).

Option 1	Option 2
1/2 c oatmeal	1 whole bagel
1 slice rye toast	1 orange
1/2 grapefruit	1 c skim milk
1 c skim milk	1/2 oz fat-reduced
1 tsp margarine	cream cheese

Option 3	Option 4
French toast:	1 whole English muffin
2 slices bread	3/4 c fresh blueberries
1 egg, whipped	1 c nonfat plain yogurt
1/4 small honeydew	2 tsp peanut butter
melon	
1 c skim milk	
1 tsp margarine	
1 tbsp syrup	

LUNCH OPTIONS

Each of these lunches provides about 500 calories from the following food groups: 2 starch servings, 1 fruit serving, a single 2-oz serving of lean meat, 1 skim milk serving, 1 vegetable serving, 1 fat serving.

Option 1	**Option 2**
Tuna pasta salad:	Chicken salad sandwich:
1 c cooked pasta	1 whole wheat pita
1 oz water-packed tuna	1/2 c diced chicken breast
1/2 c shredded carrot	2 tsp chopped celery
1/2 c zucchini, celery	1 tbsp low-calorie salad dressing
1 tbsp low-calorie Italian dressing	Raw vegetables
3 oz low-calorie frozen yogurt topped with sliced strawberries	1 medium pear
	1 c skim milk

Option 3	**Option 4**
Spaghetti and meatballs:	3 oz trimmed pork chop
1 c spaghetti	Hot mustard
3/4 c tomato sauce	3 steamed new potatoes
2 medium meatballs	French-cut green beans
1 tbsp grated Parmesan cheese	1 slice pumpernickel bread
Mixed green salad	1 tsp margarine
2 tbsp low-calorie Italian dressing	10 large green grapes
1/2 c fruit salad	

Option 3	**Option 4**
Ham sandwich:	Individual pizza:
2 slices rye bread	1 whole English muffin
2 oz lean ham	1/4 c spaghetti sauce
2 tsp diet mayonnaise	2 oz part-skim mozzarella cheese
Tomato slices, lettuce	Tossed salad
Carrot sticks	1 or 2 tbsp low-calorie salad dressing
12 large bing cherries	1 peach
1 c skim milk	1 c skim milk

Common Considerations

Another question women have about their bodies during weight training is: What are the effects on the bustline? First, don't expect any miracles. The breast itself isn't made of muscle tissue. However, exercises for the underlying pectoralis (chest) muscles can cause an uplifting of the breasts. Additionally, exercise can lead to a loss of body fat, which could result in a reduction in bust size. Therefore, a firming effect could be achieved.

DINNER OPTIONS

Each of these dinners provides about 500 calories from the following food groups: 2 starch servings, a single 3-oz serving of lean meat, 2 vegetable servings, 1 fruit serving, 1 fat serving.

Option 1	**Option 2**
3 oz broiled halibut	Fajita:
Baked potato, small	2 oz chicken breast, sautéed with green pepper, onion
1 tbsp low-calorie sour cream	Top with salsa and 1 oz low-fat cheddar cheese
Steamed broccoli with lemon	Fold into large flour tortilla
Kiwi and raspberries	
Whole wheat dinner roll	Cauliflower/broccoli medley
1 tsp margarine	1 c assorted fruit chunks
Coffee or tea	

TRAINING FOR SENIORS AND ADOLESCENTS

Particular groups of women need special care, and these unique needs must be considered when designing strength training programs. The older woman and the adolescent young woman need some adjustment of their strength training programs to ensure safety and effectiveness.

Seniors.

In recent years, exercise scientists and gerontologists have begun to emphasize the importance of muscular fitness for older people. Impaired muscle functioning has been linked to many problems in older adults, especially women. For instance, the typical 75-year-old woman often doesn't have enough muscle strength in her legs to rise efficiently from a seated position, walk, or maintain her balance. The long-range implication is that independent living will no longer be possible for many older women.

If you are an older woman, an appropriate strength training program can help your overall functioning and well-being. Strength training

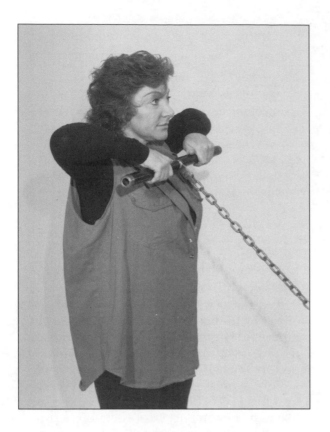

programs for your leg fitness can lead to improvements in your balance and walking and can reduce your potential for falling. Strength training also will offer you greater self-confidence and feelings of self-worth. While the thought of "pumping up" might seem strange to you, it is clear that an appropriate level of muscle strength is needed for you to remain healthy and independent.

Osteoarthritis. Many experts believe that strength training can also help you effectively manage osteoarthritis. Your ability to live with osteoarthritic changes depends on how the stresses around your joints are shared by the surrounding muscles and unaffected joints. Stronger muscles can absorb more of the attendant stress on a joint, thereby reducing the stress placed on the affected joint surfaces.

Osteoporosis. Osteoporosis, an age-related disorder affecting many older women, is characterized by a decreased bone mineral content. It has been positively influenced by strength training. There is evidence showing that resistance exercise slows bone loss and can increase bone density. When muscle-movement stress is applied to the bone, the pressure produces a desirable response by the bone. Training-induced improvements in muscle strength and balance may help prevent falls that cause many fractures among elderly osteoporotic women.

Muscle tissue. Strength training also can help you preserve muscle tissue as you age. Muscle tissue is more metabolically active than fat tissue (it will burn more calories). By maintaining more muscle tissue throughout your life, you will also maintain a higher metabolic rate throughout your life and will have an easier time maintaining your optimal body weight.

Strength training guidelines. There are few daily activities that don't require some muscular fitness. By doing a sound strength training program you are more likely to maintain appropriate muscular fitness and a higher level of functioning. As a result, you will be more able to perform your normal activities and maintain an independent lifestyle.

An appropriate strength training program for you as an older woman should include following the guidelines and principles discussed in the subsequent chapters. These are the most important factors to remember:

- Focus your strength training program on developing enough muscle function to live a physically independent lifestyle.

- Learn the proper techniques for all the exercises in your program.

- Maintain your normal breathing patterns while exercising, because holding your breath can cause blood pressure elevations.

- Control the speed of all the exercises. To prevent orthopaedic trauma to your joint structures, don't do any fast or jerky movements.

- Never participate in strength training exercises during active periods of arthritic pain because exercise could make this condition worse.

- Control the range of motion so that you exercise through the maximum range of motion that doesn't cause pain or discomfort.

- Never use a resistance that is so heavy you can't do at least 8 repetitions per set. Heavy resistances can be damaging to your skeletal and joint structures; therefore, every set should consist of 8 to 12 repetitions for all strength training exercises.

- As you get stronger, achieve an overload first by increasing the number of repetitions and then by increasing the weight lifted.

- Limit each of your workouts to one or two sets of 8 to 10 different exercises; the selection of exercises should include all your major muscle groups.

- Don't overtrain. Two sessions per week are needed to get a positive physiological response. Depending on the circumstances, more sessions may not be desirable or productive.

- Do multi-joint exercises (as opposed to single-joint exercises) because they will help you develop functional strength.

- Given a choice, use machines to strength train, rather than free weights. Most machines require less skill, allow you to start with lower resistances and increase by smaller increments, and more easily control the exercise range of motion.

- Your first several strength training sessions should be closely monitored by a trained professional who is sensitive to the special needs and abilities of seniors.

Common Considerations

Another question women ask is: How can I use my mind to enhance my strength training efforts? You'll see tremendous results simply from making up your mind to strength train—making a commitment and sticking to it. Using your mind to keep your motivation up is another way to help your efforts. Visualize yourself meeting your goal. If you want to be able to carry heavy loads without getting tired, picture yourself doing it. If your goal is to trim down so you'll look magnificent in your summer bikini, picture yourself on the beach, wearing your suit, and looking dazzling. Some women use their minds to concentrate on each muscle as they exercise. They visualize it working and growing. Using your mind to relax after a workout also can be helpful. Relaxation enables the body to rest—time during which it will repair itself and heal.

Adolescents.

Not long ago the prevailing attitude in the medical community was that adolescents shouldn't be allowed in strength training programs because of their young age. Their concerns were the safety issues relating to strength training for the pre-

teen population. These concerns addressed three issues: whether strength gains were possible, whether youths (male and female) benefited from strength training programs, and how strength training programs for youths should be designed. Fortunately, these questions stimulated research that led two major organizations (American Academy of Pediatrics and National Strength Coaches Association) to develop position papers making recommendations about adolescents (defined here as young women between the ages of 11 and 13) and strength training. The efforts of these professional groups have prompted further research on the matter.

Research has shown that strength training, when properly performed, can be a productive (the benefits far outweigh the risks) endeavor for girls. Youngsters can get many benefits from participating in a sound, supervised strength training program. Some desirable results are improved muscle strength, better local muscle endurance, stronger connective tissue resulting in increased resistance to injury, enhanced motor performance in certain sport activities, and a greater appreciation of the value of fitness. De-

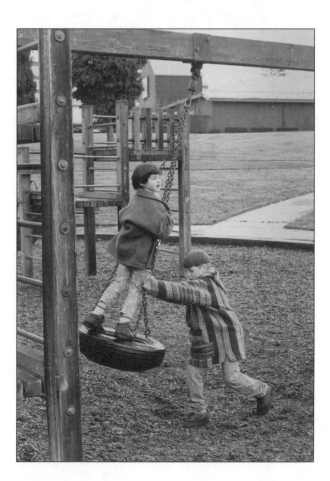

spite its many beneficial aspects, strength training for youths is not without risks. Of greatest concern is the potential for damage to the developing skeleton and supportive tissues of the adolescent.

Strength training can be a safe and productive exercise for young women. Yet, it is necessary to take precautions to guarantee that nothing done will place a young woman's developing musculoskeletal system at risk. Perhaps the two most important factors for strength training to be a safe, effective, and enjoyable activity for young women are quality supervision and adherence to the concept of minimum effective dosage (MED). Design the training program using only the minimum effective dosage of resistance exercise needed to produce a training effect.

The following principles are suggestions to those interested in developing a sound strength training program for adolescents. In many instances, these guidelines are similar to those for the elderly because the need for following safe and effective practices while exercising transcends age.

- No matter how big, strong, or mature a young woman appears, remember that she is physiologically immature.

- Make sure that every young woman is taught and uses proper breathing techniques and proper training techniques for all of the exercise movements involved in the program.

- Stress that speed should be controlled in all exercises. To prevent orthopaedic trauma to the joint structures, no fast or jerky movements should be allowed while exercising.

- Under no circumstances should a weight be used that allows less than 8 repetitions to be completed per set. Heavy weights can be damaging to the developing skeletal and joint structures. Each set of an exercise should consist of 8 to 12 repetitions. Although you should ensure that adolescents train hard and are challenged, it is not recommended that they exercise to the point of momentary muscle fatigue.

- As a training effect occurs, achieve an overload first by increasing the number of repetitions, and then by increasing the weight.

- Perform one or two sets of 8 to 10 different exercises; the selection of exercises should include all the major muscle groups.

- Do two strength training sessions per week.

This is enough because young women need, and should also do, other forms of physical activity.

- Perform full range, multi-joint exercises (as opposed to single-joint exercises), because they facilitate the development of functional strength.

- Don't overload the skeletal and joint structures of the adolescents with maximal weights. This is particularly dangerous to the preteen whose skeletal system is highly prone to orthopaedic trauma, because of the presence of active growth plates (areas where cartilaginous tissue is being converted to hard, bony tissue).

- Finally, and perhaps most importantly, closely supervise all strength training activities with appropriately trained personnel.

Common Considerations

Another question women have is: What effect will strength training have on my sleep patterns? When beginning a strength training program, some women will notice a need for more sleep. Then, as their bodies strengthen, their need sometimes decreases. Overall, aim for 7 or 8 hours of sleep. If you find that you're always tired, you may need a change in your program (as mentioned in chapter 2), or your diet may need a boost.

TRAINING DURING AND AFTER PREGNANCY

Of the many questions about exercise and pregnancy, one that is frequently raised is: Can women safely do strength training during pregnancy? The responses to this question are varied, largely because of the lack of information about strength training and pregnancy. Many women would like to continue their strength training during pregnancy but are confused by the diverse opinions on the subject. In recent years, several well-respected members of the medical community and exercise scientists have developed specific guidelines for pregnant women interested in strength training.

Based on the limited data available, most experts agree that proper strength training poses little risk to either the mother or the developing fetus. In fact, strength training may be beneficial for the pregnant woman. Strength training should provide the pregnant woman with the muscle strength needed for the postural adjustments that occur during pregnancy. The maintenance of improved posture should help diminish a pregnant woman's low back pain (a very common occurrence in pregnancy). Daily activities should also be easier for the pregnant woman with improved muscle strength.

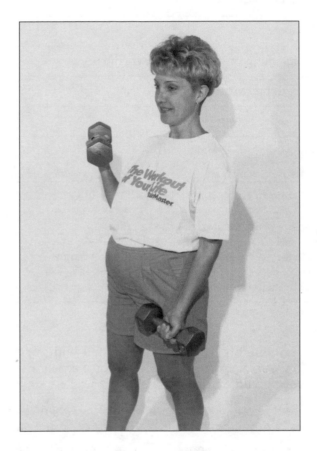

Limited research has shown that strength training can be part of a balanced exercise program for a pregnant woman. Strength training may help you manage many rigors of pregnancy more effectively. Research also suggests that strength training may not be appropriate for every pregnant woman. Until more data is available, each pregnant woman should consult her physician for advice. In addition, training programs for those pregnant women who do strength training should be individualized. People who design strength training programs for pregnant women should be conservative in manipulating the training variables. Research suggests that the following recommendations for strength training and pregnancy are appropriate:

- If you have health and medical conditions that can place you or the fetus at risk, you should not participate in strength training during pregnancy (see Table 1.1).

- If you have never participated in a strength training program, you should not begin one during pregnancy.

- No ballistic exercise movements should be used. During pregnancy, you experience increased joint and ligament laxity, raising your susceptibility to soft tissue injury.

- You are encouraged to breathe normally during exercise, because oxygen delivery to the placenta may be reduced if you hold your breath while exerting force.

- You should avoid maximal lifts and heavy resistances because they may expose your joint and skeletal structures to excessive forces. An exercise set of at least 10 repetitions will ensure that resistances aren't too great.

- As you get stronger, it is recommended that overload be achieved first by increasing the number of repetitions and then by increasing the weight lifted.

- You should do one set of 8 to 10 different exercises two times per week, involving all of your major muscle groups.

- Strength training machines are generally preferred over free weights because they require less skill and can be more easily controlled.

- If a particular exercise produces pain or discomfort, stop it and do an alternate exercise.

- You should immediately consult your physician if any of the following warning signs or complications appear: vaginal bleeding, abdominal pain or cramping, ruptured membranes, elevated blood pressure or heart rate, or lack of fetal movement.

POSTPARTUM WOMEN

Not long ago, women were instructed to stay in bed for up to 2 weeks following an uncomplicated delivery. Fortunately, medical professionals now know better. It is now accepted that the sooner you get moving, the better off you are. Exercise—particularly specific strength activities—can help you tone your saggy abdominal region, improve your posture, and regain your prepregnancy shape.

Table 1.1 Medical Conditions Considered Risky for Strength Training During Pregnancy

Absolute risks	Relative risks
Heart disease	High blood pressure
Ruptured membranes	Anemia or other blood disorders
Premature labor	Thyroid diseases
Multiple gestation	Diabetes
Bleeding	Palpitations or irregular heart rhythms
Placenta previa	Breech presentation in the last trimester
Incompetent cervix	Excessive obesity
History of 3 or more spontaneous abortions or miscarriages	Extreme underweight
	History of precipitous labor
	History of intrauterine growth retardation
	History of bleeding during present pregnancy
	Extreme sedentary lifestyle

Several physical changes occur shortly after you've given birth to that beautiful little boy or girl. Your hormonal levels change to help your uterus, cervix, and birth canal contract and to prepare your body for lactation.

Certain exercises should be started soon after you've given birth. Most physicians will instruct their patients to perform Kegel exercises almost immediately after the delivery. Kegel exercises, named after the physician who devised them, help keep your vagina elastic and prevent you from having bladder problems. To do Kegel exercises, you simply pretend that you are stopping and starting your urine flow. The muscles you exercise by performing Kegel exercises help you control your bladder and support the contents of your abdomen.

The day after your delivery (provided it was uncomplicated), your physician may recommend that you do pelvic tilts to strengthen and tone your abdominal muscles. During your pregnancy these muscles can become stretched to hold the growing fetus. Pelvic tilts will also help you re-lieve the low back strain associated with carrying your baby. To properly perform a pelvic tilt you should do the following:

- Lie on your back with your knees bent and your hands relaxed by the side of your head.

- Tighten the muscles of your lower abdomen by tilting your pelvis rearward and flattening your lower back against the floor.

- Hold this position for 5 to 10 seconds, relax, and repeat 8 to 12 times.

Before you do more vigorous strength training activities during the postpartum period, you should consult your physician. Your body will take several weeks to heal following labor and delivery. Episiotomies and vaginal tears take time to heal. The point of attachment between the placenta and your uterus needs healing time. Recovery rates differ from woman to woman, birth to birth, and typically take between 6 weeks and 3 months. Your physician is the best judge of when you can safely resume vigorous exercise.

CHAPTER 2

ORGANIZING YOUR PROGRAM

You've identified your goals; it's time to develop a plan and put that plan into action. This chapter will help you develop a strength training program that will—within the parameters of your unique situation—enable you to achieve and maintain your objectives.

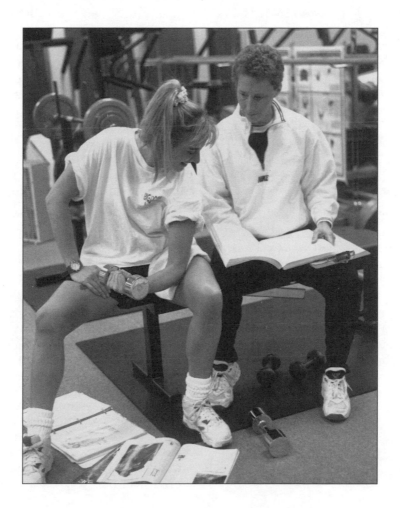

DEVELOPING YOUR PLAN

Once you've decided your goals, the next step is to design a program to meet them. Designing a strength training program involves seven variables:

- Selecting your exercises
- Ordering your exercises
- Determining repetitions
- Determining sets
- Determining weight
- Limiting the time between exercises
- Allowing time between your workouts

SELECTING YOUR EXERCISES

As a rule of thumb, you should limit your workout to 12 to 14 exercises. Doing more than 14 exercises is counterproductive physiologically and psychologically. You reach a point where additional work is not worth the effort. Your workout should include about 10 exercises that will develop the major muscle groups in your body (lower back and buttocks, legs, torso, arms, and abdominals), plus 2 to 4 exercises chosen to meet your particular needs or interests. For example, if you're prone to groin pulls, you'll want to include exercises for your inner thigh muscles. If you're a tennis player, you may want to include exercises for your forearms—the gripping muscles.

ORDERING YOUR EXERCISES

Strength training programs should begin with exercises using the largest muscles and move to those using the smallest muscles. Most strength training exercises are designed to develop the largest muscle involved in the exercise. If you stop an exercise because a smaller muscle has become fatigued before a larger one, then you've compromised the possible gains for the larger muscle. For example, if you start your workout with modified sit-ups, you'll fatigue your abdominal muscles—muscles that should be exercised last. A problem then occurs when you do an exercise (such as a squat) in which your abdominals act as stabilizers. You have to either lift less weight during the exercise (decrease your need for stabilization), or subject yourself to risk of injury (exercise at a level of intensity that your abdominals can't safely support). Either way, you may lose.

DETERMINING REPETITIONS, SETS, AND WEIGHT

These three variables are the numbers crunch of strength training. A repetition is doing a specific exercise one time. A set is doing a particular number of repetitions in a row, before stopping. The weight used is the level of resistance (demand) that you put on your muscles while exercising. You have many choices about how to structure your repetitions, sets, and weight. We'll present two: the multiple- and single-set approaches.

Multiple-Set Approach.

The traditional approach to strength training suggests that you

- complete three sets of 5 to 8 repetitions for developing strength, or
- complete three sets of 9 to 15 repetitions for developing endurance.

When taking the traditional approach, use a weight that will enable you to do all sets somewhere between the minimum and maximum number of repetitions before reaching muscle failure (inability to complete a repetition). Or select a weight based on the "one-max rep system" by determining the maximum amount you can lift in one repetition of an exercise, and then lift an arbitrary percentage of that amount on each set of the exercise.

Single-Set Approach.

Another popular, yet less traditional, approach to strength training is high intensity training (H.I.T.). H.I.T. proponents believe that "more is *not* better." They claim that once you work your muscles to their capacity, additional work is a waste of time and possibly counterproductive. H.I.T. involves performing one set of 8 to 12 repetitions until you reach muscle failure, whether you're developing strength or endurance. In other words, you should lift a weight that will let you do at least 8, but not more than 12, repetitions of the exercise. You should increase the amount you lift when you can do 12 repetitions. If you can't do 8 repetitions at the increased weight, you've increased the weight too much.

Individuals who support the H.I.T. approach believe that most people don't have a constant maximum strength. Your mental state can greatly affect how much you can lift. If you're "up," you often feel like you can lift the world. If you're "down," you may feel like every weight is attached to a Wurlitzer piano. Unfortunately, it is sometimes difficult to determine what mental state you're in. If you do your best on every exercise and follow sound training guidelines, you'll achieve positive results.

Strength training practitioners disagree about which approach (multiple-set or single-set) produces the best results. Given our experiences at West Point and in the corporate world, we advocate the single-set H.I.T. theory. We witnessed wide success with this philosophy. It quickly produced great results, generally established an environment that led to increased exercise adherence, and kept the number of injuries to a very low level. We recognize, however, that adopting a training philosophy is best left to each individual. If you feel that the multiple-set program for training is appropriate for you, follow that approach.

LIMITING THE TIME BETWEEN EXERCISES

Limit the time between exercises to less than one minute to make the most of your time in the weight room. No science involved here, just sound time management. Minimize your standing around. Get in and get out without chaos or wasted time. Minimizing the time between exercises helps you focus on maximum effort while you're training.

ALLOWING TIME BETWEEN YOUR WORKOUTS

Unless you are doing a split routine workout (upper body exercises one day, lower body exercises the next day), allow at least one full day between workouts. An alternate-day schedule (Monday-Wednesday-Friday or Tuesday-Thursday-Saturday) is the most commonly followed system. As you get older, you need more rest between workouts. You may want to occasionally give yourself two full days of rest between workouts instead of one.

ASSESSING YOUR STRENGTH

Once you have your strength training plan it's time to get a "status report" about your level of strength and endurance. Assessing your level of muscular fitness can help you see where to begin your strength program and what deficiencies

you might have, such as weak abdominals, a low level of upper body strength, or strong quadriceps but weak hamstrings. Then your training program can be tailored to take care of these issues.

Muscle strength is usually assessed by devices for measuring muscle strength and endurance or by calisthenic tests. Most testing with devices is conducted in a laboratory because they often require trained personnel to use and are relatively expensive. If you are interested in such high-tech evaluation, your local fitness center will either have the equipment or have someone who can tell you about a nearby testing locale.

For most of us, calisthenic tests are appropriate for assessing our upper body strength and endurance, and they can be done in almost any setting (including at home). This type of testing usually needs little or no equipment, allows more than one person to be tested at a time, and involves functional body movements. Calisthenic tests measure how well you can do calisthenic exercises, such as push-ups, sit-ups, pull-ups, and dips. When you perform a calisthenic test, you determine the maximum number of repetitions you can successfully complete. One of the more commonly used calisthenic tests is the modified push-up.

The modified push-up begins with a warm-up by stretching your shoulders and triceps (see Figure 2.1).

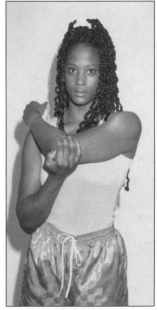 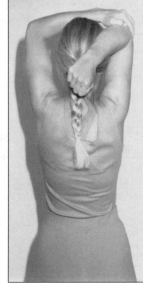

Figure 2.1a   Shoulder stretch.   **Figure 2.1b**   Triceps stretch.

Place yourself on the floor so that your body is straight and your weight is on your hands and knees (see Figure 2.2). Be sure your hands are flat on the floor and directly under your shoulders. Lower your chest until it touches the floor, then push yourself back up to the starting position. Exhale each time you push your body up; do not hold your breath. Keep your body straight, and fully straighten your arms at the end of each push-up. Count "one" each time you do a push-up correctly, and stop the test when you must rest. (Note: despite its widespread use in testing, the modified push-up is not nearly as effective for muscular conditioning as negative-only push-ups, see page 94.) Record the number of push-ups you could do and compare your score to the standards in Table 2.1. You can perform a similar test for your abdominal muscle strength. Standards for sit-ups appear in Table 2.2. You should

be pleased if you are in the average or high categories, but don't be discouraged if you are below average or low—you've just taken the first step to improve your strength.

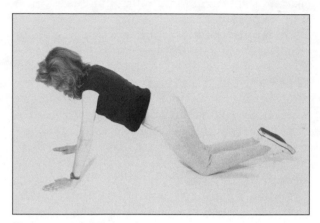

Figure 2.2   Modified push-up.

Table 2.1   Muscular Fitness Norms (Modified Push-Ups)

	Score at age				
	20-29	30-39	40-49	50-59	60+
High	34+	25+	20+	15+	5+
Average	17-33	12-24	8-19	6-14	3-4
Below average	6-16	4-11	3-7	1-5	1-2
Low	0-5	0-3	0-2	0	0

Note. Adapted by permission of Macmillan Publishing Company from *Health and Fitness Through Physical Activity* by M.L. Pollock, J.H. Wilmore, & S.M. Fox. Copyright © 1978 (New York: Macmillan Publishing Company).

Table 2.2   Muscular Fitness Norms (Modified Sit-Ups)

	Score at age				
	20-29	30-39	40-49	50-59	60+
High	39+	31+	26+	21+	16+
Average	33-38	25-30	19-25	15-20	10-15
Below average	29-32	21-24	16-18	11-14	6-9
Low	0-28	0-20	0-15	0-10	0-5

Note. Adapted by permission of Macmillan Publishing Company from *Health and Fitness Through Physical Activity* by M.L. Pollock, J.H. Wilmore, & S.M. Fox. Copyright © 1978 (New York: Macmillan Publishing Company).

Assessing your strength also can be important after you've started your program. Testing can help evaluate the progress you're making in your program. For example, if you do the push-up test and find that you're not showing improvement in the number of push-ups you can do correctly, you may need to adjust your exercise routine. On the other hand, if you find that you've improved your strength, you'll be motivated to continue exercising. Positive feedback from your exercising can support your attitudes toward the value of your efforts.

LEARNING THE BASICS

You should become familiar with the training principles to make sure you get the most out of your strength training sessions.

INTENSITY

A muscle becomes stronger when a demand is placed on it. If you place less demand than your muscles can handle, then you'll get less improvement than you are capable of achieving. If you do a biceps curl set using a 10-lb dumbbell for six consecutive workouts, you won't get as much improvement as if you had increased your weight to 12 or 15 lbs after the third workout—making your workout more *intense*. Practitioners debate about what level of intensity you need to achieve maximum results. We believe that anything less than an all-out effort will produce less than maximum gains. Another theory suggests that an appropriate demand is achieved by training at a predetermined percentage of your maximum for each exercise. Depending on your philosophy, the percentage may change from set to set and from exercise to exercise.

SPECIFICITY

Only one proper way exists to perform a specific exercise, and you should emphasize correct technique when strength training. If you compromise the mechanics for an exercise, you will compromise the results. Learn how to do each exercise, and then do them all correctly. (See chapters 4 to 7 for explanations of how to perform the exercises most often used in strength training programs.) Keep in mind that how you do an exercise is much more important than how much weight you lift. One of the most effective ways to

make sure you use the proper techniques is to work out with a training partner who knows how to perform the exercise and who has the temperament to help you train correctly.

Specificity also involves selecting the right exercise to develop each muscle. If you want to develop a specific area of your body, you need to know what exercises will help you do this. Table 2.3 illustrates what exercises are used for the major muscle areas of the body. Sample training programs for developing specific areas of your body appear in chapter 10.

PROGRESSION

Your strength training program should be progressive in nature. Too much, too soon will lead either to an injury or failure, or both. You should gradually increase the stress on your muscles as they are able to meet the demand. As they can handle the stresses imposed on them (by getting stronger), you should gradually increase the resistance level to stimulate new growth and development.

RECOVERY TIME

When you stress a muscle beyond what it can normally handle, some rest is needed for the muscle tissues, tendons, and ligaments to recover. If the time between exercise sessions is too brief, your muscle may be unable to make the adaptations needed before being stressed again. In this instance, the muscle either will not develop to the extent possible or may suffer a decrease in strength. Conversely, if you take too much time between workouts, your muscles will gradually return to their untrained level.

MINIMIZING INJURY, MAXIMIZING RESULTS

Doing your strength training exercises properly will give you results more quickly and efficiently, and ensure you are safe from injuries. In the following discussions we'll show why proper technique is crucial, how to achieve it, and how to ensure your safety.

MUSCLE BALANCE

You have muscles that oppose each other—your quadricep muscles (front thigh) are opposed by your hamstring muscles (rear thigh). If one is too

Table 2.3a   Strength Training Exercises for Selected Muscles

Lower body muscles	Exercises*			
	Free weights	Multistation machine	Variable resistance machines	Buddy/stick exercises
Back	Barbell Squat Barbell Dead Lift Stiff-Legged Dead Lift	Back Extension	Back Extension	Leg Press (buddy)
Buttocks	Barbell Squat Barbell Dead Lift	Leg Press	Back Extension Leg Press Hip Abduction	Leg Press (buddy) Hip Abduction (buddy)
Front thighs	Barbell Squat Barbell Dead Lift Dumbbell Step-Up Dumbbell Lunge	Leg Extension Leg Press	Leg Extension Leg Press Hip Abduction	Leg Press (buddy)
Back thighs	Barbell Squat Barbell Dead Lift		Leg Curl Leg Press	Leg Curl (buddy) Leg Press (buddy)
Hip flexors	Dumbbell Step-Up Dumbbell Lunge			Hip Flexion (buddy)
Calf muscles	Barbell Heel Raise		Heel Raise	Heel Raise (buddy)
Inner thigh			Hip Adduction	Hip Adduction (buddy)
Outer thigh			Hip Abduction	Hip Abduction (buddy)

*We recommend that you perform abdominal curls/crunches or bent-knee modified sit-ups for training your abdominal muscles.

Table 2.3b Strength Training Exercises for Selected Muscles

Upper body muscles	Exercises			
	Free weights	**Multistation machine**	**Variable resistance machines**	**Buddy/stick exercises**
Shoulder	Dumbbell Upright Row Bench (Chest) Press	Upright Row Bench (Chest) Press	Arm Cross Seated Row Seated Press	Bent-Arm Fly (buddy) Front Raise (buddy) Bent-Over Side Lateral Raise (buddy) Lat Pulldown/Shoulder Press (stick)
Upper back	Dumbbell Upright Row Dumbbell Shoulder Shrug	Upright Row Shoulder Shrug	Seated Press Seated Row	Shoulder Shrug Back Pulldown/Bench (Chest) Press (stick) Bent-Over Side Lateral Raise (buddy)
Side	Dumbbell Bent-Over Row	Lat Pulldown	Pullover	Lat Pulldown/Shoulder Press (stick)
Chest	Bench (Chest) Press	Bench (Chest) Press	Arm Cross	Bent-Arm Fly (buddy) Front Raise (buddy)
Biceps	Dumbbell Bent-Over Row Dumbbell Biceps Curl	Upright Row Biceps Curl Lat Pulldown	Biceps Curl	Biceps Curl (stick) Lat Pulldown/Shoulder Press (stick) Back Pulldown/Bench (Chest) Press (stick)
Triceps	Bench (Chest) Press	Triceps Extension Bench (Chest) Press	Seated Dip	Triceps Extension (stick) Lat Pulldown/Shoulder Press (stick)
Forearm flexors and extensors	Wrist Curl Reverse Wrist Curl	Wrist Curl Reverse Wrist Curl		

strong for the other, you risk injury to the weaker muscle. Pairs of opposing muscles should have about a 1:1 strength relationship. The exception is your quadriceps and hamstrings, which should be 3:2 (your quadriceps should be about 150% stronger than your hamstrings). For maximum results, alternate pushing exercises with pulling exercises (do a leg press, then a leg curl). A complete workout routine that alternates pushing and pulling exercises appears in chapters 4 to 7.

FULL RANGE OF MOTION

Every exercise should be done through a full range of motion (the degree to which there is movement around a joint). If you don't go through a full range of motion, you will perform less work and eventually will decrease your flexibility in the joints involved in the exercise.

SPEED OF MOVEMENT

Do every exercise at a controlled speed. If you raise and lower a weight slowly (about 2 seconds on the lifting phase and 4 seconds on the lowering phase), your muscles will do effective work throughout the exercise. If you throw or jerk the weight, your muscles will be working only at the beginning and at the end of the lift. No work will be done in the midrange of the lift. Additionally, the rapid deceleration in throwing a weight increases your chances of being injured.

SAFETY CONSIDERATIONS

Among the factors involved in resistance training *none* is more important than safety. In addition to using the proper lifting techniques we have outlined, follow these safety principles: warm up properly, handle muscle soreness effectively, use well-trained spotters, breathe properly, wear appropriate clothing, and use correct grip positions. If you adhere to these guidelines and use common sense, strength training is a relatively safe activity.

Warming up. Common sense suggests that you spend a few minutes before strength training to prepare for the demands of rigorous activity. Warming up serves several purposes. The primary purpose is to slowly elevate your pulse to an aerobic level, increasing your cardiac output. As a result, your body and muscle temperature is raised. This increases the activity of the enzymes in the working skeletal muscles, which increases the metabolism of those muscles. The

viscosity in the muscle is reduced, and muscle blood flow is increased. Therefore more oxygen and fuel reach the muscles involved in the activity.

A proper warm-up improves the mechanical efficiency and power of the working muscles. The time necessary to transmit nervous impulses is also improved, augmenting your reaction time and coordination. Warming up decreases the likelihood of injuries to the muscles and the supporting connective tissues involved in the activity. The increase in temperature and blood flow to these muscles and supporting tissues is particularly beneficial if you are doing high-powered, explosive exercises.

A warm-up session should be at least 5 minutes, raise the core temperature of your body (signaled by perspiration), and involve your major joints. A typical warm-up session might include running in place (see Figure 2.3) for a minute and then doing a set of strength exercises using very light resistance.

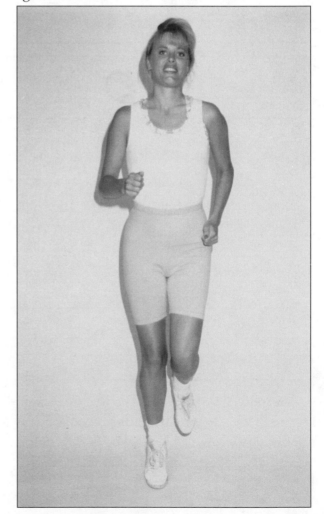

Figure 2.3   Running in place.

Muscle Soreness. There are several different theories about the cause of muscle soreness that persists for 2 or 3 days after an unusually hard strength training workout. The most widely accepted theory is that it results from microtears to the muscle and its tendinous attachments. Usually this damage occurs during the beginning of a program when the relatively understressed muscle fibers haven't adapted to the new demands. Soreness also can occur when you dramatically increase the intensity of your training or incorporate new exercises.

Spotters. Spotters help you while you are doing resistance training. Their assistance can take many forms. Their job is to ensure that you are not injured by having a weight fall on you. If you can't complete a repetition, your spotter will take the weight from you, if asked. Spotters can also get help if you are injured while training. Another purpose of spotters is to give you constant verbal feedback—either to motivate you or to ensure that you use the proper techniques. Spotters can help you bring a heavy weight into the starting position for an exercise (particularly for negative-only training). Remember, anyone with the responsibility of spotting must know the proper techniques in the exercises you're performing.

Breathing. Never hold your breath while strength training. Holding your breath while exerting force can cause a dangerous buildup of inner-thoracic pressure. The pressure inside your rib cage compresses the right side of your heart. This restricts the flow of blood and, consequently, oxygen to your entire body (a process called the "Valsalva maneuver"). Two theories are generally advocated concerning the proper approach to breathing while strength training. The simplest and most sensible guideline suggests that you should breathe normally and regularly as you train. A second and more involved theory contends that you should control your breathing pattern while you exercise. Proponents of this theory recommend that you inhale during the negative (lowering) phase of the exercise and exhale during the positive (lifting) phase of the exercise.

Proper clothing. Perspiring is your body's primary mechanism to prevent overheating. When you exercise and your internal temperature rises, your body's thermal control systems activate. Blood travels through the exercising muscle and picks up heat in the process. The blood is brought close to the skin and you perspire. The perspiration evaporates as it contacts the atmosphere. The cooled blood then travels back through your body, reducing your core temperature. You should wear comfortable, loose-fitting clothing that allows the air to cool your skin. Wearing a rubber sweat suit, for example, prevents cooldown and can result in heat injury or even death.

Grips. When you train with free weights, you can use one of four grips to hold a barbell: overhand, underhand, alternate, and false (see Figure 2.4).

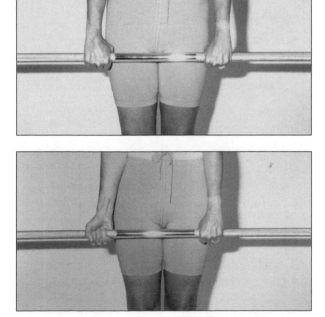
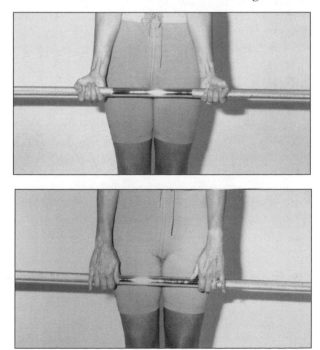

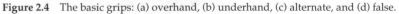

Figure 2.4 The basic grips: (a) overhand, (b) underhand, (c) alternate, and (d) false.

The most widely used grip is the overhand grip. In this grip, your thumbs are hooked underneath the bar with your knuckles on top of the bar. For an underhand grip, the opposite is true—your thumbs are hooked over the bar, while your knuckles are underneath the bar. An alternate grip combines the overhand and the underhand grips. One of your hands is above and the other hand is below the bar. Of the four grips, the alternate is the strongest. In a false grip your thumbs are not hooked around the bar, and you substitute comfort for safety. This grip is not recommended for beginners.

Vary the width of your grip depending on the exercise you are doing and what's comfortable for you. The width of your grip should provide maximum range of movement, isolation of the muscle(s) being exercised, and comfort. Whatever grip you use for a particular exercise, use it every time you do that exercise.

FINE-TUNING YOUR EFFORTS

As you progress through your strength training program, you will notice many changes in how you look, feel, and perform. You also might notice that, although you've been working out consistently, a particular muscle has reached its peak—you just can't seem to lift more weight. Maybe you'll find that you're not as interested in strength training as you used to be, or that your muscles are getting unusually sore. Conversely, perhaps you've "caught fire" and want to lift for power or for competition. We'll show you how to deal with these issues in the following discussion.

STRENGTH PLATEAUS

During a strength plateau, further gains in strength in a muscle or muscle group have temporarily halted. For whatever reason, you can't make progress on a particular exercise; you can't handle more resistance. Normally a plateau doesn't occur in all muscle groups at the same time. If you're stuck for more than a few consecutive workouts, you can use one or more of the following techniques for overcoming a strength plateau:

- Include different exercises in your program.
- Change the frequency of your training.
- Change the number of sets you perform.

- Modify your exercise—do more repetitions with less resistance or fewer repetitions with more resistance.
- Increase the intensity level of your workouts.

OVERTRAINING

Design your program so that it gives enough training stimulus for positive physiological changes without going beyond your abilities. Overtraining occurs when there is an imbalance between training and recovery. The symptoms of overtraining vary from one person to another. The most common signs frequently involve one or more of the following:

- Chronic muscle or joint soreness
- Increased incidence of musculoskeletal injuries
- Impaired physical performance
- Reduced enthusiasm and desire for training
- Increased resting heart rate (your heart rate taken first thing in the morning, before rising out of bed)
- Increased resting blood pressure
- Increased incidence of colds and infections
- Impaired recovery from exercise (you remain highly fatigued well after you finish your workout)
- Increased perceived exertion during your normal workouts
- Reduced appetite
- Undue weight loss
- Disturbed sleep patterns
- Increased depression, irritability, or anxiety

DETRAINING

Detraining occurs when you cease or reduce your training efforts. This can lead to losses in strength and other benefits you may have achieved in a strength training program. To maintain gains in strength, the intensity of demand on your muscles must be kept at least at the existing program levels. However, you can reduce the volume and frequency of your training without appreciably affecting your level of strength.

COMPETITIVE RESISTANCE TRAINING

Competitive resistance training has become extraordinarily popular. The number of women in the three most popular resistance training sports—bodybuilding, power lifting, and Olympic lifting—is increasing every day. Bodybuilding is a sport that involves developing a physique emphasizing size, symmetry, and definition. Power lifting involves determining who, in a particular weight class, can lift the most total weight in three distinct lifts—the bench press, squat, and dead lift. Olympic lifting involves determining who, in a particular weight class, can total the most weight for two combined lifts: the snatch, and the clean and jerk.

POWER

Many competitive sports involve some degree of power—a frequently misunderstood physical component. Power is simply the rate at which work is performed. In strictly scientific terms, it is the amount of work performed over a given period of time, as expressed by the following equation:

$$Power = \frac{Work}{Time}$$

Because work, by definition, is the application of force through a range of motion (distance), power can be expressed as the product of force times distance divided by time, or as the product of force times velocity (velocity = distance divided by time). This equation is expressed as:

$$Power = \frac{(Force \times Distance)}{Time}$$

or

$$Power = Force \times Velocity$$

It should be clear from these equations that while speed and strength are important components of power, they are not the same as power. Muscle power is dependent on the interaction of speed, distance, and strength. Power can be improved through resistance training by increasing

- the speed of muscle contraction,
- the distance of muscle contraction, and
- the strength of muscle contraction.

Record Keeping

Record what training you performed during every workout: what exercises you did, in what order you did them, how many sets and reps of each you did, how much resistance you used, and any other relevant information (injuries, unusual events that may have affected your workout, etc.). Use your log to accomplish these objectives:

- Adjust future workouts.
- Increase the intensity of your training session.
- Measure your improvement.
- Identify weaknesses in your training program.
- Help motivate you to continue exercising.

EVALUATING YOUR WORKOUT

Strength is usually equated with lifting a set amount. How often have you heard, "She can bench press 125 lbs"? Such reliance on the number of pounds you can lift can lead to injury, disappointment, and failure to reach your training goals.

Once you realize that how much weight you lift is not always an accurate measure of how much work you do, you will be on your way to getting the most from your efforts. An easy way to assess your efforts is to look at three perspectives:

- How much is much?
- How much is possible?
- How much is enough?

HOW MUCH IS MUCH?

If asked about how much work they did in their strength training workouts, most women would measure their effort in absolute terms. They lifted and lowered a specific amount of weight, a given number of times. If asked about how strong they are, most women who are seriously into lifting would probably answer in terms of a maximum effort on a common lift, such as the bench press. This is the basis of their inclusion in such performance clubs as the "humongous-poundage" bench press club. Seldom does anyone involved realize that earning membership in such a group has more to do with genetic factors, such as the length of the lifter's limbs, than it does with strength.

How you lift (proper training technique) is more important than how much. Concentrating on how much can lead to frustration, injuries, staleness, or abandonment of your strength training efforts.

How Much Is Possible?

Several factors affect how strong you can become. How much you lift is influenced by at least seven factors:

- The intensity of your strength training program
- Your predominant muscle fiber type
- Your hormonal levels
- Your body proportions
- Your muscle insertion points
- Your muscle-tendon ratios
- Your neurological efficiency

Except for the intensity of your exercise, the other factors are beyond your control. They are genetically predetermined. Although you can't alter the genetic cards "dealt" to you at birth, you can get stronger. You should train hard and be content with the results. How much is possible? The answer will be known only after you've engaged in a proper program of strength training.

How Much Is Enough?

The key to knowing how much is enough involves shifting your focus from the numbers game and redirecting your efforts. If you want to maximize your benefits in the weight room, focus your attention on developing functional strength. Functional strength is the degree of muscle strength required to perform daily tasks (including leisure activities) without undue fatigue or risk of injury. How much is enough? At a minimum, you should train at a level that will give you the quality of life you desire and deserve.

Now that you've mastered the basics, let's look at strength training equipment and other factors to consider when selecting your workout environment.

CHAPTER 3

WEIGHING YOUR OPTIONS

One advantage of using strength training to meet your workout goals is that you can tailor your program to meet your needs. You have many choices about what equipment and what environment is best for you.

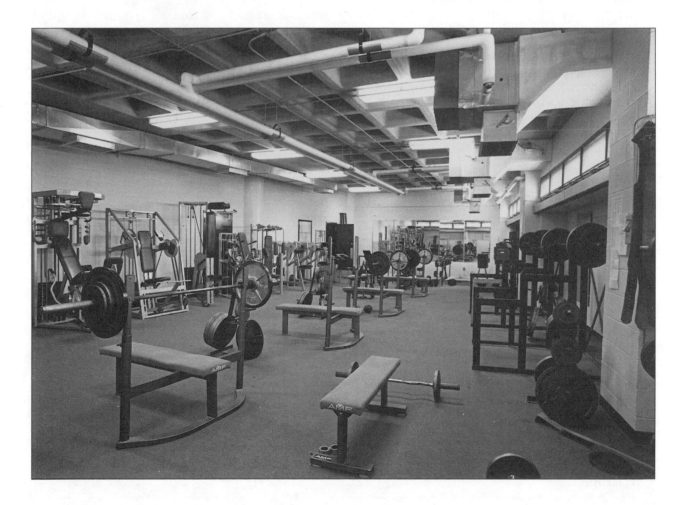

SELECTING YOUR EQUIPMENT

A variety of equipment is available to help you reach your strength training goals. Some is more expensive. Some is more complex. Some requires more skill to use. Some is more time efficient. Some is more safe. Almost all of this equipment can enable you to meet your training goals.

Like most people, you might not have access to all the commonly used types of strength training equipment. If you do, you may be uncertain about what equipment is best for you. The basic guideline to follow when selecting your equipment is to choose what will best meet your interests and needs. At the minimum, select equipment that is readily accessible (compatible with your workout schedule, requires a minimum of travel inconvenience, etc.) and is consistent with your personal preference.

If you have a choice of strength training equipment, one approach is to list the advantages and disadvantages of each type and then make your subjective decision. Table 3.1 compares four types of equipment on selected criteria. We'll discuss each type in detail.

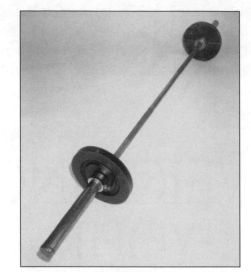

Figure 3.1a   Exercising with a barbell.

FREE WEIGHTS

Free weight equipment for strength training includes barbells and dumbbells (see Figure 3.1). A standard barbell is a bar that is usually 60-84 in. long and can vary in both weight and diameter. Weights are attached to the ends of the bar

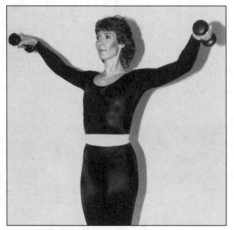

Figure 3.1b   Performing a side lateral raise with a dumbbell.

Table 3.1 Comparing Strength Training Equipment				
	Free weights	Multistation machines	Variable resistance machines	Buddy/stick exercises
Cost	Low	Somewhat high	High	Very low
Functionality	Excellent	Limited	Limited	Excellent
Learning curve	Limited	Excellent	Excellent	Variable
Muscle isolation	Variable	Excellent	Excellent	Excellent
Rehabilitation	Excellent	Excellent	Excellent	Excellent
Safety	Relatively safe	Very safe	Very safe	Very safe
Space efficiency	Variable	Excellent	Variable	Excellent
Time efficiency	Variable	Excellent	Excellent	Excellent
Variety	Excellent	Limited	Limited	Excellent
Versatility	Excellent	Limited	Limited	Excellent

to provide resistance. The weight is secured to the bar with either fixed collars (the amount can never be changed) or adjustable collars (you can put whatever amount you want on the bar each time you train). Fixed collars offer the advantages of safety (the plates can't slip off while you're lifting), time efficiency (you don't have to adjust the amount of weight), and neatness (weight plates aren't scattered about). Adjustable collars enable you to adjust the amount of weight on the bar to your personal needs.

A dumbbell is a short barbell (8 to 14 in. long). Similar to a barbell, weights are attached to the ends of the dumbbell to provide a resistance. The weights may be either fixed, as on most dumbbells, or adjustable. Holding a dumbbell in each hand, you can perform many exercises that can be done with a barbell. Dumbbells offer several advantages: they enable you to strengthen both sides of your body equally; they enable you to do some exercises (like a side lateral raise) that can't be done with a barbell; they add variety to your workout; and they let you exercise one side of your body even if the other side is injured or immobilized and cannot be trained.

Depending on your interests and personal philosophy, free weights offer several advantages over other equipment. When compared with machines, their primary advantage is that people of all sizes can use them. When using free weights to train specific muscle areas, just change your hand and foot placement. Free weights offer a greater variety of exercises than other equipment, and they easily enable you to identify a weakness or muscle imbalance. If one side is weaker than the other, you won't be able to lift the weights evenly (one side will come up before the other). Free weights allow you to train functionally—they enhance joint stability and encourage your muscles to work in concert. Finally, free weights are relatively inexpensive and require little upkeep.

In addition to barbells and dumbbells, your free weight equipment can include curl bars, benches, abdominal boards, lifting platforms, and squat racks. A curl bar (see Figure 3.2) is a bar shaped

specifically to increase the efficiency of the biceps curl exercise. It does this by placing your hands and biceps in a more biomechanically comfortable position while you train. Lifting benches (see Figure 3.3) enable you to vary the position of your

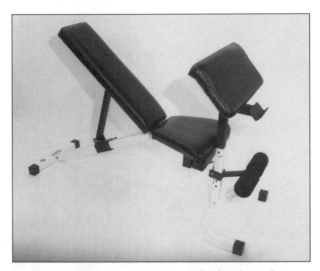

Figure 3.3a   Incline bench with a preacher bench attachment.

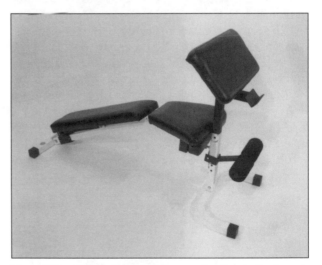

Figure 3.3b   Decline bench with a preacher bench attachment.

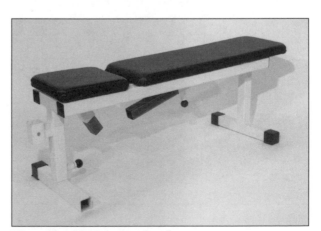

Figure 3.3c   Multi-purpose bench.

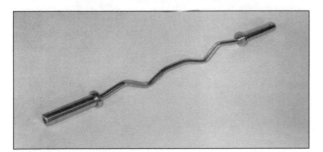

Figure 3.2   A curl bar.

Table 3.2   Strength Training Benches

Type of bench	Adjustable	Purpose
Power bench	No	A bench that is used primarily to perform the bench press exercise.
Incline bench	Some are adjustable	This bench (which rests at an inclined angle) inclines your body while training. For example, a 45-degree inclined angle is midway between the position for doing a bench press and the position for doing a standing overhead press.
Decline bench	Some are adjustable	This bench lays flat and is used primarily when performing a decline bench press to place a greater demand on the lower region of the chest muscles.
Multipurpose bench	Yes	This bench adjusts for both decline and incline and is used for most exercises involving a bench.
Preacher bench	No	This bench helps to isolate the biceps muscle while performing the biceps curl exercise.

body while you exercise so that muscles can be either isolated or trained at a specific angle. Table 3.2 describes some commonly used benches.

An abdominal board (see Figure 3.4) is a platform that enables you to exercise your abdominal muscles in a variety of angles and positions. A lifting platform is a platform you stand on while you exercise. It helps to prevent damage to the floor if you drop the weights after an overhead lift. A squat rack (see Figure 3.5) solves the problem of lifting heavy weights from the floor to your shoulders during the squat exercise.

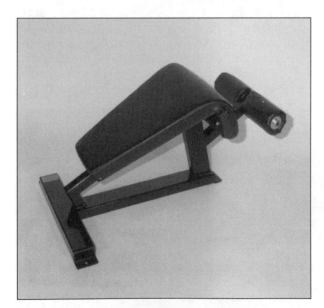

Figure 3.4   An abdominal board.

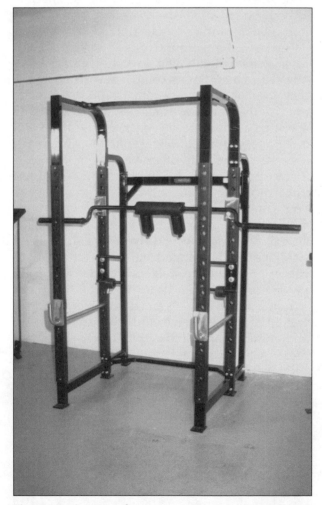

Figure 3.5   A squat rack.

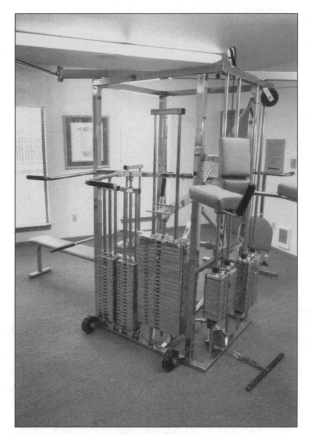

Figure 3.6   A multistation machine.

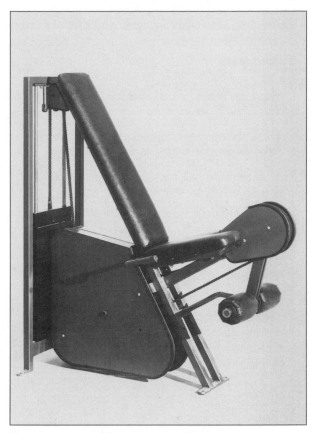

Figure 3.7   A variable resistance machine.

MULTISTATION MACHINES

A multistation machine has several exercise stations that collectively can serve many people at once (see Figure 3.6). Although different manufacturers make this type of equipment, people often refer to it by the name of the company that pioneered the multistation machines—Universal Gym.

Multistation machines are so versatile that you can use them for most of the exercises you do with barbells. They also enable you to do some exercises that you can't do with barbells, such as leg extensions, leg curls, and lat pulldowns. A multistation machine offers several advantages, including a high level of safety (particularly when compared to free weights); an ability to accommodate several people simultaneously in a small space; a high degree of time efficiency (little time is needed to use the pin-operated weight stacks); a quick learning curve (such machines are very easy to operate); and a variable resistance capability in some of the more recently developed machines.

VARIABLE RESISTANCE MACHINES

Depending on your body position at different stages while you exercise, you are stronger at some points and weaker at others. For example, the biceps muscle is weakest at 100° and strongest at 60° in the range of motion for the arm curl exercise. Variable resistance machines (see Figure 3.7) adjust for these differences as you exercise. Nautilus, Eagle, and Keiser machines are examples of equipment that vary the resistance.

The primary advantage of variable resistance equipment is that it enables you to develop each muscle to its fullest potential throughout the range of motion. It also encourages you to work through a greater range of motion, which provides a very safe way to train, and enables you to exercise at or near your fatigue threshold. The main disadvantage of this type of equipment is its higher cost.

Table 3.3   The Advantages and Disadvantages of Using Low-Cost Equipment

Advantages	Disadvantages
• These exercises permit many people to train simultaneously.	• Both buddy exercises and stick exercises require two people—an exerciser and a partner. You may not always have a training partner available at a convenient time.
• These techniques allow you to do many different exercises for developing strength.	• For some people, these techniques may be harder to learn than doing exercises on a machine that is designed to control the movement pattern.
• In most instances, these techniques permit you to control how fast you perform an exercise.	• For a few people, these techniques may require more coordination than what is needed with traditional strength equipment.
• Properly performed, these exercises permit your muscles to be worked at a very high intensity (i.e., to the point of momentary muscle fatigue).	• Buddy exercises and stick exercises aren't as effective when one partner is much stronger or taller than the other. The ability of the weaker or shorter person to apply enough resistance can be limited by strength or leverage deficiencies.
• These exercise techniques can rechannel your focus away from how much work you are doing (quantity) to the more critical issue—how well you are working (quality).	• These techniques don't offer feedback about how much work is being done. Some people prefer knowing they've lifted "X" number of pounds, "X" number of times.

LOW-COST EQUIPMENT

All factors considered, free weights don't involve much expense (in comparison to machines). Several effective alternatives for developing strength exist that don't require much, if any, equipment. For example, until the mid-1970s, most of the strength training equipment for the United States Military Academy was bars with cement-filled coffee cans secured to the ends. Remember that to develop muscular fitness, you have to take one basic step—place a demand on the muscle or muscle group you want to improve. How you accomplish that is based on many factors—not the least of which is your ingenuity. The advantages and disadvantages of using low-cost equipment appear in Table 3.3. Four of the most effective low-cost techniques for developing muscular fitness are: negative-only exercises, buddy exercises, stick exercises, and resistance cord exercises.

Negative-Only Exercises.

These are based on the principle that the muscles you use to raise a weight are the same muscles you use to lower (under control) the weight. When you lift a weight, your muscles are shortening. When you lower a weight (the negative phase of the lift), your muscles are lengthening.

Negative-only exercises are calisthenics that use only the negative phase of the exercise. The most common negative-only exercises are push-ups, dips, chin-ups, pull-ups, and sit-ups. In a negative-only push-up, you do that part of the exercise in which you slowly lower yourself to the ground. You don't push yourself back up to the starting position. You can increase the difficulty of the exercise by taking longer to lower yourself or by wearing a weighted vest. To do another repetition, you repeat the process.

Buddy Exercises.

You do these exercises against force exerted by a partner. Buddy exercises (see Figure 3.8) are also called manual resistance exercises (MREs) and partner resistance exercises (PREs), and have been used since the early 20th century to develop strength. In recent years buddy exercises have been used extensively by the military and by professional and intercollegiate athletic teams for developing and maintaining muscle strength.

Buddy exercises can be used to develop a variety of the muscles in your body. For example, to do a buddy exercise for developing your abductor muscles you would lie on your side. Slowly raise your upper leg (the one away from the floor) against resistance applied by your buddy. Your partner should apply enough force to enable you to complete the movement in 2 or 3 seconds (see Figure 3.8).

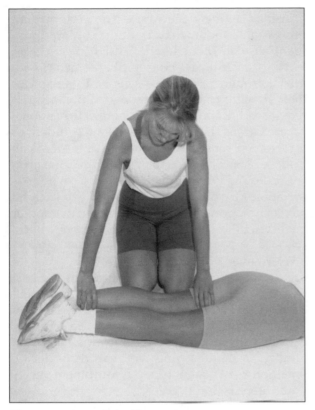

Figure 3.8   A sample buddy exercise.

Stick Exercises.

Stick exercises are buddy exercises designed to develop your upper body strength. They use a wooden dowel (see Figure 3.9) or some other cy-lindrical device, such as a broomstick or a base-ball bat. This wooden dowel provides an added degree of comfort and control. The conditioning program at the United States Military Academy uses a 30-in. wooden dowel to do stick exercises. At the minimum, the dowel should be as long as the width of the exerciser's shoulders.

Stick exercises usually involve combining two movements into one exercise. Among the more popular stick exercises are: the lat pulldown/shoulder press, the chest press/lat row, the biceps curl/negative curl, and the triceps extension/negative extension. To do a lat pulldown/shoulder press stick exercise, begin in a seated position with your arms extended, shoulder-width apart, over your head. Your partner stands behind you and places a knee against your back to support you. Your partner then places the dowel in your outstretched hands and holds the dowel next to your hands. On command, pull the dowel downward to the base of your neck against resistance provided by your partner (this movement is a lat pulldown). Pause momentarily and push the dowel back to the starting position against force exerted by your buddy (this phase of the exercise is a shoulder press). To do another repetition, repeat the process.

Resistance Cord Exercises.

Resistance cord exercises involve doing exercises against the force required to stretch a cord or to return it to its natural state. Cords must be made of elastic materials like rubber (see Figure 3.10). A resistance cord can be either a commercial product or a homemade device, such as a length of surgical tubing. Resistance cord exercises can be done for both the lower body and the upper body. Begin either by attaching one end of the cord to a fixed object or by holding one end with

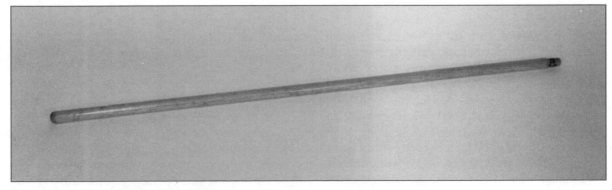

Figure 3.9   A dowel used for stick exercises.

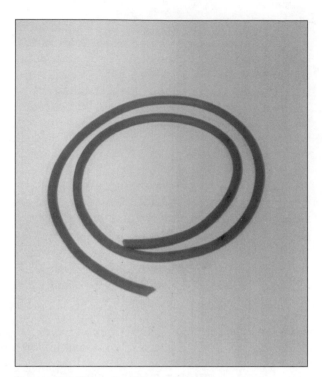

Figure 3.10   Using a stretch cord for resistance exercises.

each hand. Then stretch the cord by moving your arm or leg in a pattern appropriate to the muscle or muscle group you want to develop.

DETERMINING YOUR WORKOUT ENVIRONMENT

As you decide what equipment to use in your strength training program, consider these six factors: where you plan to train, professional advice you have received, the specific exercises your program requires, safety, cost, and personal preference. Weigh the importance of each factor and then reach your decision.

TRAINING LOCALE

If you plan to strength train at home, you have considerable control over what equipment you use (subject to cost and space limitations). Most people, however, train in facilities outside their homes—health and fitness clubs, schools, YWCAs, work, and the like. If you have a choice of workout facilities, take stock of what strength training equipment each facility has—you'll want to use equipment that meets your specific needs and interests. Most larger health and fitness clubs have a mix of free weights and machines, but

some facilities, for philosophical, space, or cost reasons, have only one type of strength equipment. Check, too, to see that the facility has enough equipment that it will be available at the time of day you want to use it.

PROFESSIONAL ADVICE

Consider getting some advice from a competent professional about what strength training equipment to use. Most health and fitness clubs, YMCAs, and colleges now employ someone with a background in exercise science to supervise their strength training facilities. (Many facilities require certification by one or more of the national organizations that set standards and guidelines for exercise prescription, such as the American College of Sports Medicine, American Council on Exercise, and the National Strength Coaches Association.) If your facility doesn't have such an advisor, try contacting a professional at another facility or the conditioning coach from a local school.

Whomever you solicit advice from, keep in mind that several theories exist about the best way to strength train. Strong feelings regarding a particular system of training may translate into similar attitudes about equipment. So carefully consider any advice you receive; don't accept it blindly. In the end, only you can truly decide whether a particular type of equipment meets your interests and needs.

PROGRAM REQUIREMENTS

You can develop each of the major muscles in your body using exercises based on various pieces of equipment. If your choices of equipment are limited, the exercises you can perform will be limited as well. If you have several types of equipment available, your range of choice is much broader. Because a few exercises can only be performed using specific equipment (for example, power lifts can only be done with free weights), you will have to have access to the necessary equipment if you want to include them in your program.

SAFETY

Machines are generally safer than free weights. Because a machine's resistance mechanism and frame are an inclusive unit, there is little chance of losing your balance, slipping, or falling while exercising on a machine. You also don't have to worry about weight shifting or about dropping a weight on yourself. Some exercisers also find machines easier to use than free weights. Because the techniques for using machines are less involved, they are easier to learn and to follow (particularly when you approach your fatigue threshold), and you're less likely to injure yourself because of improper technique. No equipment, though, is fail-safe. The best way to prevent injury and maximize your safety is to follow proper techniques and appropriate training principles.

Cost

Strength equipment varies widely in cost. If you plan to exercise away from home, your primary financial considerations will be the cost to join or use the facility and miscellaneous related expenses (travel, parking, etc.). If you decide to strength train at home, you probably will need to buy at least a few pieces of equipment, depending on your personalized program. But before you outfit a home gym, decide exactly what you want to accomplish in training and what equip-

ment you need to achieve your goals (within the confines of your budget and space limitations). Once you make those decisions, start looking for equipment. Get professional advice, comparison shop, and get information on guarantees and warranties. If you're not buying locally, be sure to find out costs for shipping, installation, and delivery. Ask about durability and how servicing and part replacement will be handled. It's your money, so spend it wisely.

Personal Preference

What equipment you use while strength training is, above all else, a matter of personal preference. Depending on your needs and interests, you may want to incorporate more than one type of equipment into your strength development program. Keep in mind that the "quality" of your training, not the type of equipment, is the critical factor in developing your muscular fitness. The best equipment in the world will do little for your muscular fitness if it is not used properly.

PART

II

LEARNING THE EXERCISES

n the following chapters you'll find exercises for free weights, multistation machines, and variable resistance machines. We'll also show you how to train using low-cost equipment. This chapter includes information on negative-only, buddy, and stick exercises.

For each exercise, we'll tell you the major muscles that are strengthened, explain the starting position, and talk you through the exercise. We'll help you ensure proper technique by emphasizing special points and including illustrations.

At the end of each chapter, we present four sample workouts for each type of exercise. Use these workouts as a framework to design a program to fit your needs. The first sample workout exercises your muscles from largest to smallest. The second emphasizes the alternation of pushing and pulling exercises. The third is a pre-exhaustion workout that will challenge your endurance and your strength. The fourth workout involves a training routine that alternates between upper and lower body exercises.

What follows is a list of the exercises you'll find in each chapter.

Frec Weight Exercises
  Barbell Squat
  Barbell Dead Lift
  Stiff-Legged Dead Lift
  Dumbbell Lunge
  Dumbbell Step-Up
  Barbell Heel Raise
  Dumbbell Bent-Over Row
  Dumbbell Shoulder Shrug
  Dumbbell Upright Row
  Dumbbell Side Lateral Raise
  Dumbbell Front Shoulder Raise
  Dumbbell Fly
  Bench (Chest) Press
  Dumbbell Biceps Curl
  Dumbbell Triceps Extension
  Wrist Curl
  Reverse Wrist Curl

Multistation Exercises

Leg Press
Leg Extension
Leg Curl
Back Extension
Lat Pulldown
Shoulder Shrug
Upright Row
Bench (Chest) Press
Biceps Curl
Triceps Extension
Wrist Curl
Reverse Wrist Curl

Variable Resistance Exercises

Back Extension
Leg Press
Leg Extension
Leg Curl
Hip Abduction
Hip Adduction
Heel Raise
Arm Cross
Seated Row
Seated Press
Pullover
Side Lateral Raise
Biceps Curl
Seated Dip
Abdominal Curl

Strength Training Without Equipment

Negative-Only Push-Ups
Negative-Only Chin-Ups
Negative-Only Dips
Negative-Only Sit-Ups
Leg Press (buddy)
Leg Curl (buddy)
Hip Abduction (buddy)
Hip Adduction (buddy)
Hip Flexion (buddy)
Heel Raise (buddy)
Front Raise (buddy)
Bent-Arm Fly (buddy)
Internal Rotation (buddy)
External Rotation (buddy)
Bent-Over Side Lateral Raise (buddy)
Back Pulldown/Bench (Chest) Press (stick)
Lat Pulldown/Shoulder Press (stick)
Shoulder Shrug (stick)
Biceps Curl (stick)
Triceps Extension (stick)

CHAPTER 4

FREE WEIGHT EXERCISES

The basic requirement for developing strength in a muscle is to place a demand on it. For dynamic strength, the muscle must perform movement against resistance greater than what it is normally exposed to. Free weights—barbells and dumbbells—provide a constant resistance throughout the range of motion of an exercise (although a given barbell or dumbbell may feel heavier in one position and lighter in another because your muscles and bones act as a lever system). Every free weight exercise has a "sticking" point—the point that determines whether you can or cannot lift a given weight. Once a weight is moved past the sticking point, less muscle effort is needed to complete the lift. Consequently, a free weight exercise produces varying levels of stress to the muscle at different points in the range of motion. Despite this limitation, free weight exercises remain a popular form of strength training.

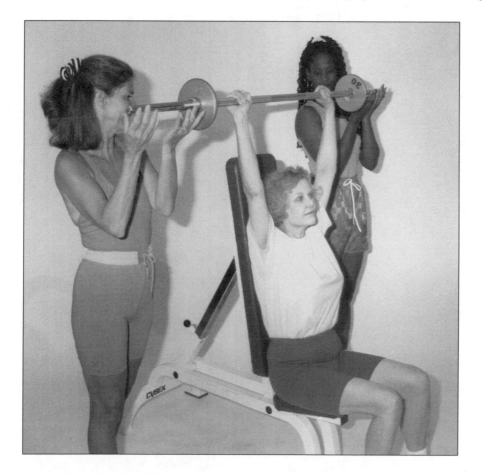

BARBELL SQUAT

Muscles used: Gluteus maximus, quadriceps, hamstrings, spinal erectors.

Starting position: Stand with your feet about shoulder-width apart and the barbell resting on your shoulders and trapezius (upper back). Do not "lock out" your legs.

Description: Slowly lower your buttocks until your thigh is parallel to the floor. Pause, then slowly recover to the starting position.

Points to emphasize:

- Keep your head up and your back straight.
- Do not bounce at the bottom of the movement.
- If needed, use heel supports, such as $2\text{-}\frac{1}{2}$-lb plates, until your ankle flexibility increases.
- Always use spotters or a safety rack when performing this exercise (not shown in photographs).
- If you find it uncomfortable to have the barbell rest across your shoulders, hold a dumbbell in each hand instead.

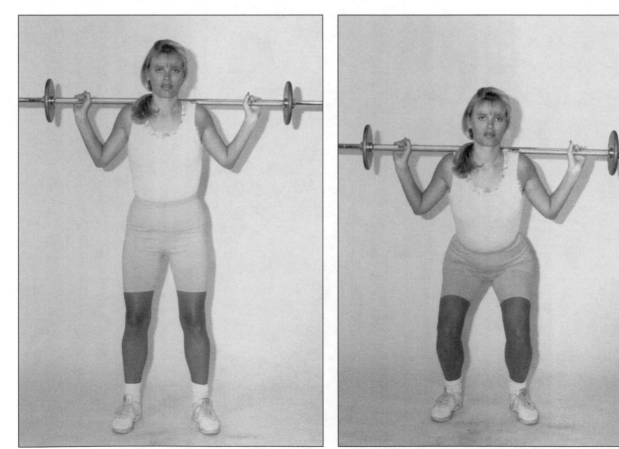

BARBELL DEAD LIFT

Muscles used: Spinal erectors, gluteus maximus, quadriceps, hamstrings.

Starting position: Stand with your feet slightly more than shoulder-width apart. Squat and grip the bar using an underhand grip with your nondominant hand and an overhand grip with your dominant hand (an alternate grip). Keep your arms straight with your elbows outside your knees and your head up.

Description: Pull the bar, while simultaneously straightening your legs and your back, until you are standing straight with your shoulders back. Pause, then slowly recover to the starting position and repeat.

Points to emphasize:

- Keep your back straight, and lift with your legs.
- Start with the bar close to your shins.
- Roll your shoulders back at the completion of the positive movement.

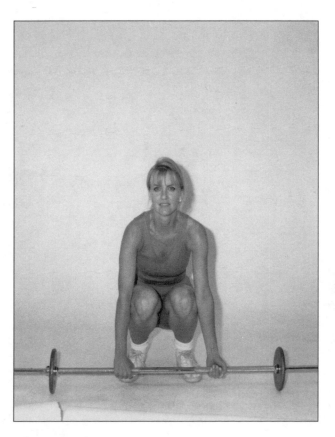
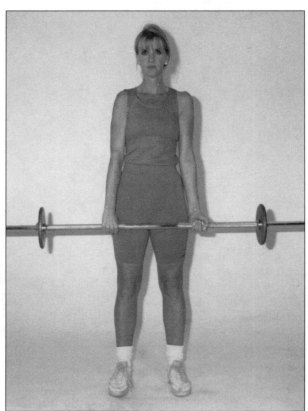

STIFF-LEGGED DEAD LIFT

Muscles used: Spinal erectors, hamstrings, buttocks, calves.

Starting position: Place your feet about shoulder-width apart (no wider). In the standing position, take the bar in your hands with an alternate grip.

Description: Bend at your waist, and lower the weight to its lowest possible point. Hang a few seconds. Pause, then return to the starting position.

Points to emphasize:

- Keep your legs locked.
- Lower the weight slowly.
- If the weight touches the floor, stand on a higher platform.
- Avoid bouncing.
- If you have a history of low back problems, you should not do this exercise.

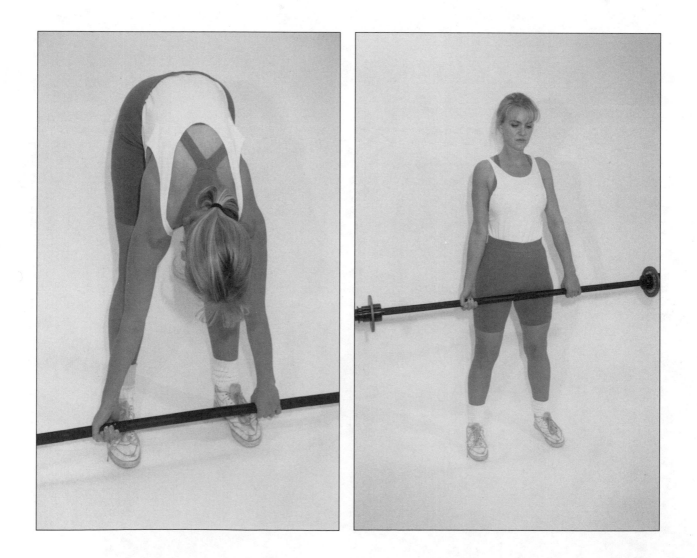

DUMBBELL LUNGE

Muscles used: Quadriceps, buttocks, hamstrings.

Starting position: Stand with your arms down at your sides, holding a dumbbell in each hand. Your feet should be comfortably together, and your head should remain erect.

Description: Stride forward with one leg. Slowly lower your body so that your upper (front) leg is parallel to the ground and your trail leg is slightly extended. Your back knee should gently touch the floor. Push back with your front leg, keeping your trunk erect. Pause, then slowly recover to the starting position. Alternate legs. Try to push with enough force to prevent your front heel from dragging on the floor.

Points to emphasize:

- Use extra caution when first learning this lift.
- Start with a light weight, learn the movement, and gradually increase the workload.

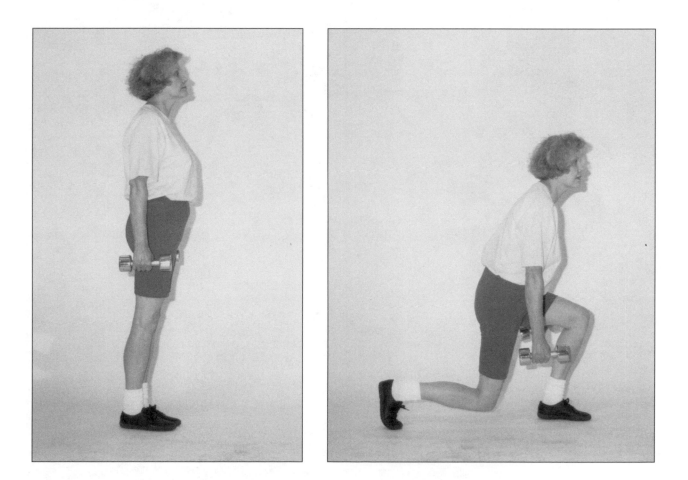

DUMBBELL STEP-UP

Muscles used: Quadriceps, buttocks, hip flexors.

Starting position: Stand with your arms extended at your sides, holding a dumbbell in each hand, similar to the lunge exercise. Your feet should be in a comfortable position.

Description: Beginning with your right leg, step up onto a bench or blocks, and lift your body with that leg. Drive the knee of your trail leg up. Slowly lower your body by stepping down, one leg at a time. Repeat, alternating lead legs.

Point to emphasize:

- Don't bounce when doing this exercise.

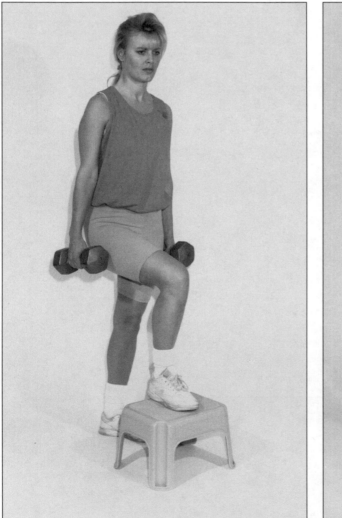
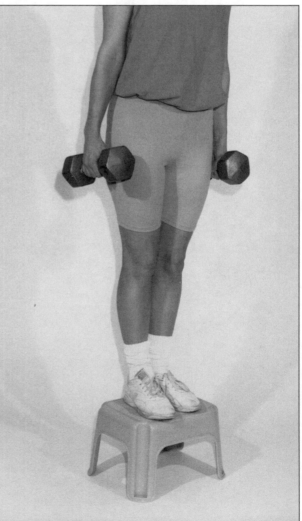

BARBELL HEEL RAISE

Muscles used: Gastrocnemius (calves).

Starting position: Stand with your toes on a piece of wood or on a barbell plate, and either place the barbell on your shoulders behind your neck or hold it using an underhand grip with your arms extended.

Description: Slowly raise your heels as high as possible. Pause, and slowly lower them back to the starting position. Upon touching the floor, immediately raise your heels again. Allow no time for rest or recovery.

Points to emphasize:

- In the starting position, place your toes in a position higher than your heels.

- Don't bounce when doing this exercise; immediately raise your heels after lightly touching the ground.

- If you find it uncomfortable to have the barbell rest across your shoulders, hold a dumbbell in each hand instead.

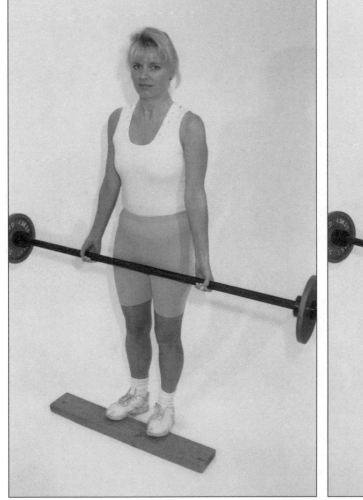
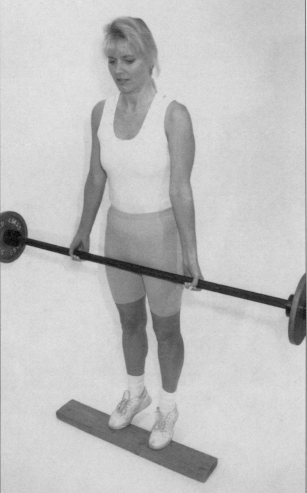

DUMBBELL BENT-OVER ROW

Muscles used: Latissimus dorsi, biceps.

Starting position: Bend forward at the waist until your torso is parallel to the floor, then place one hand on a flat bench. Grip a dumbbell with your other hand while your arm is fully extended.

Description: Slowly raise the dumbbell toward your armpit. Pause, then slowly lower the dumbbell to the starting position and repeat. Alternate arms.

Points to emphasize:

- Keep your head up and your back straight.
- Keep your back parallel to the floor.
- Don't bounce or jerk.
- Don't allow the weight to touch the floor.
- Put one hand on the bench to support your upper body and reduce the stress on your lower back.

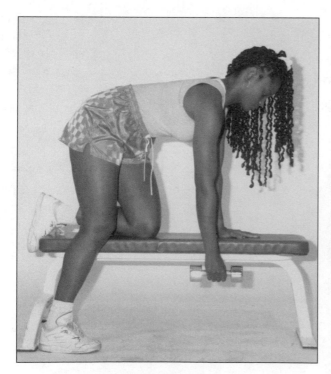 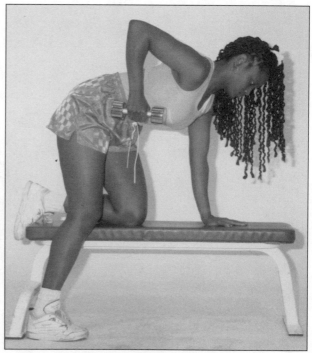

DUMBBELL SHOULDER SHRUG

Muscles used: Trapezius.

Starting position: Stand with your arms fully extended at your sides with a dumbbell in each hand.

Description: Keeping your arms straight, raise your shoulders as high as possible. Pause, then slowly recover to the starting position and repeat.

Points to emphasize:

- Stand straight.
- Allow your shoulders to drop as far as possible at the bottom of the movement.
- Don't bend your elbows to lift the weight.

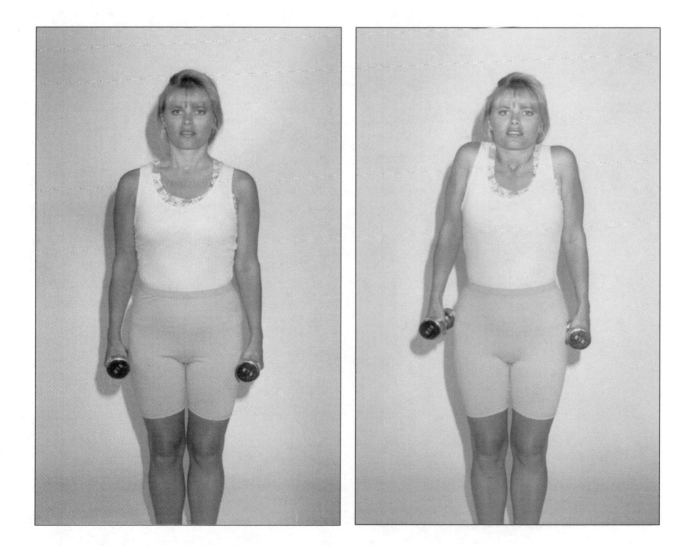

DUMBBELL UPRIGHT ROW

Muscles used: Deltoids, trapezius, biceps.

Starting position: Stand and extend your arms at your sides with a dumbbell in each hand. Use an overhand grip with your hands less than shoulder-width apart.

Description: Pull the dumbbells upward, without bending your torso, until they reach the level of your chin. Pause, then slowly recover to the starting position and repeat.

Points to emphasize:

- Stand straight with your head up.
- Pull the dumbbells all the way up to your chin.

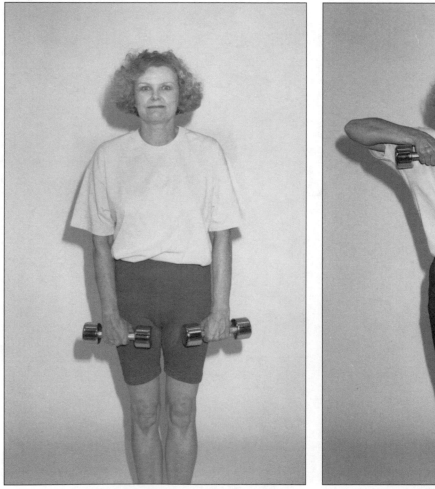 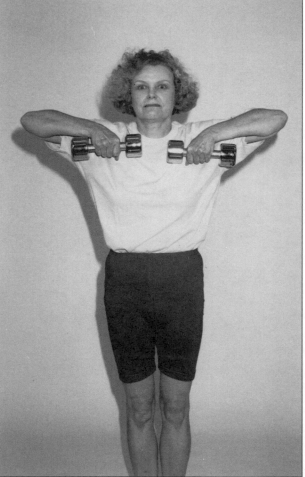

DUMBBELL SIDE LATERAL RAISE

Muscles used: Deltoids (lateral).

Starting position: Stand with your arms fully extended at your sides with a dumbbell in each hand. Your arms should hang at your sides with your elbows slightly bent.

Description: Slowly raise both dumbbells to the sides away from your body until your arms are parallel to the floor. Pause, then slowly recover to the starting position and repeat.

Points to emphasize:

- Keep your elbows slightly bent.
- Don't raise your arms any higher than parallel to the floor.

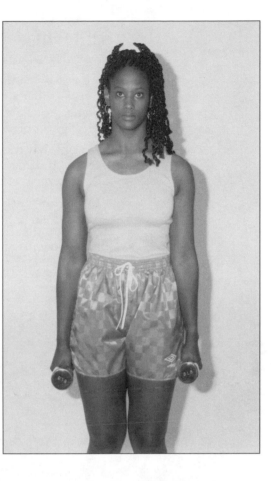

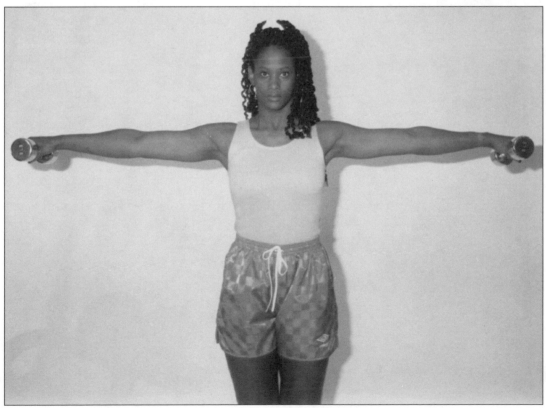

DUMBBELL FRONT SHOULDER RAISE

Muscles used: Deltoids (anterior).

Starting position: Stand with one foot in front of the other and your arms fully extended at your sides with a dumbbell in each hand. Your arms should hang at your sides with your elbows slightly bent.

Description: Slowly raise both dumbbells to the front, away from your body, until your arms are parallel to the floor. Pause, then slowly recover to the starting position and repeat.

Points to emphasize:

- Keep your elbows slightly bent.
- Don't raise your arms any higher than parallel to the floor.

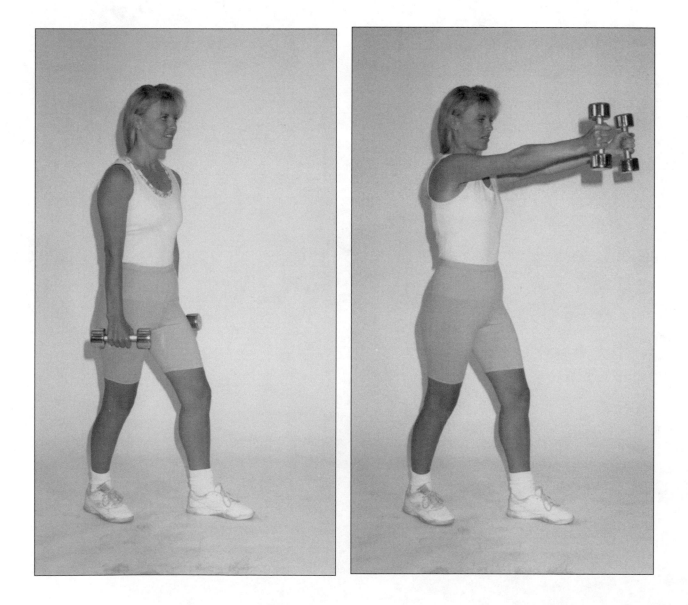

DUMBBELL FLY

Muscles used: Pectorals, deltoids (anterior).

Starting position: Lie with your back on a flat bench and your feet flat on the floor. Extend your arms upward, directly above your chest, while holding a dumbbell in each hand. Your elbows should be slightly bent.

Description: Moving your arms out toward the sides of your body, slowly lower the dumbbells toward the floor. Lower the dumbbells until they are slightly below your chest. Pause, then slowly recover to the starting position. Your elbows should remain slightly bent.

Points to emphasize:

- Maintain a slight bend in your elbow when doing this exercise.

- If necessary, use a spotter to hand you the dumbbells after you are positioned on the bench.

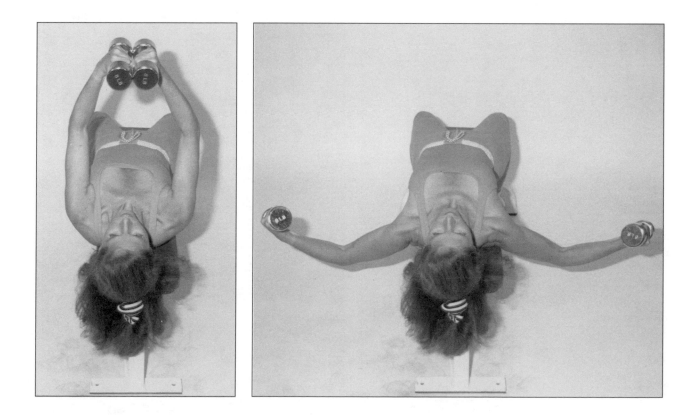

BENCH (CHEST) PRESS

Muscles used: Pectorals, deltoids, triceps.

Starting position: Lie on a bench with your feet flat on the floor. Grip the bar with your hands slightly more than shoulder-width apart.

Description: Lift the barbell from the standards and lower it to the center of your chest. Pause, then push your arms upward until your elbows are extended and repeat. Your wrists should be kept straight and directly above your elbows as you lower the bar toward your chest.

Points to emphasize:

- Use a spotter.
- Keep your head, shoulders, back, and hips flat on the bench.
- Don't bounce the weight off your chest.
- Exhale while raising the weight.

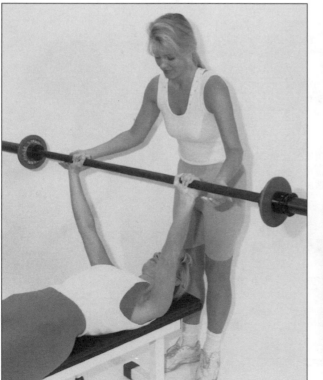
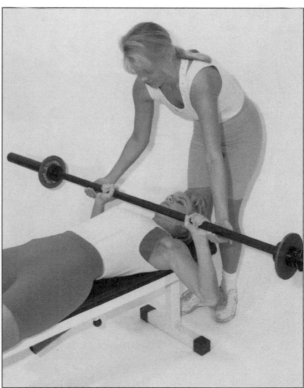

DUMBBELL BICEPS CURL

Muscles used: Biceps.

Starting position: Sit on a flat bench with your arms hanging at your sides and a dumbbell in each hand. Use an underhand grip.

Description: Keeping your shoulders fixed, curl dumbbells toward your shoulders. Pause, then slowly recover to the starting position.

Points to emphasize:

- Keep your back straight (don't lean back).
- Keep your elbows back.
- Keep your shoulders in a fixed position.

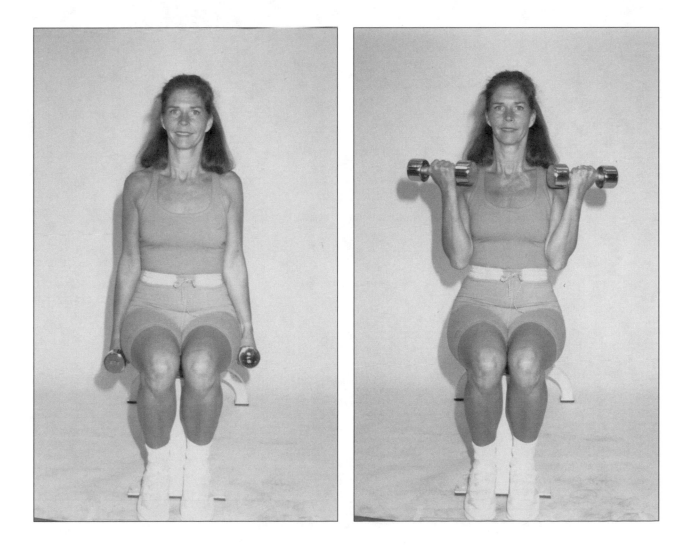

DUMBBELL TRICEPS EXTENSION

Muscles used: Triceps.

Starting position: While sitting on a bench, grasp a dumbbell between the thumbs and forefingers of both hands. Hold the dumbbell directly behind your head so your upper arms are perpendicular to the floor.

Description: Extend your arms upward until your elbows are straight and the dumbbell is directly overhead. Pause, then slowly recover to the starting position and repeat.

Points to emphasize:

- Keep your upper arms perpendicular to the floor.
- Keep your elbows shoulder-width apart.
- Keep your back straight.

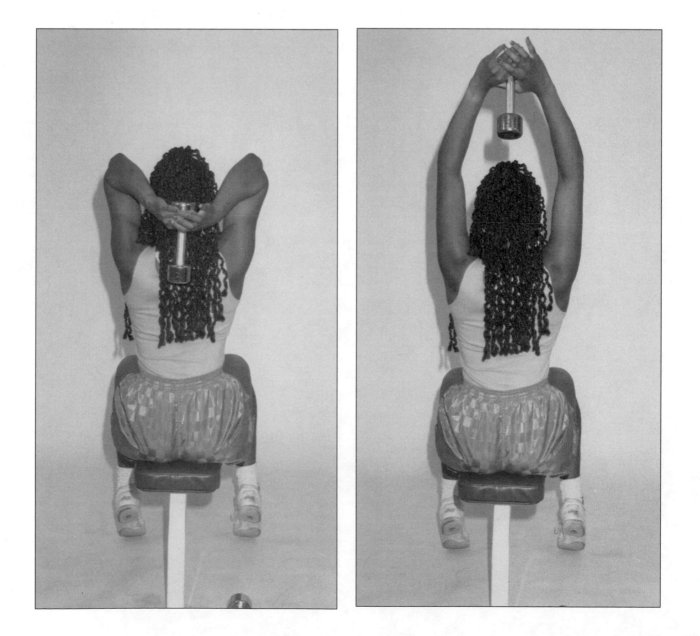

WRIST CURL

Muscles used: Forearm flexors.

Starting position: Sit on the end of an exercise bench with your forearms resting on your thighs. Grip a barbell with an underhand grip, and allow your wrists to bend downward.

Description: Curl the bar up toward your elbows as far as possible. Pause, then slowly recover to the starting position and repeat.

Points to emphasize:

- Keep your forearms flat on your thighs.
- Keep your wrists just over the ends of your knees.

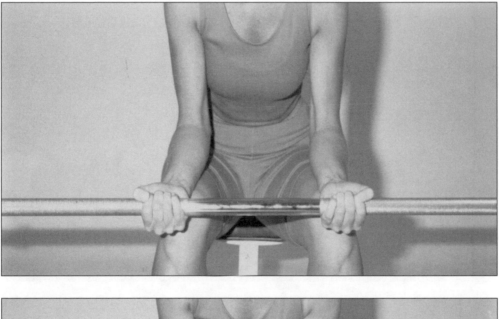

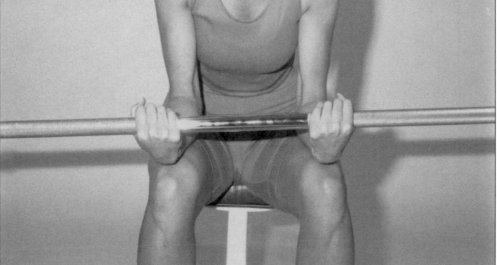

REVERSE WRIST CURL

Muscles used: Forearm extensors.

Starting position: Sit on the end of the bench with your knees bent and your feet flat on the floor. Place your forearms firmly against your thighs. Grip a barbell with an overhand grip, and allow your wrists to bend downward.

Description: Curl your wrists up and back as far as possible. Pause, then slowly recover to the starting position and repeat.

Points to emphasize:

- Keep your forearms in contact with your thighs.
- Keep your wrists just over the ends of your knees.

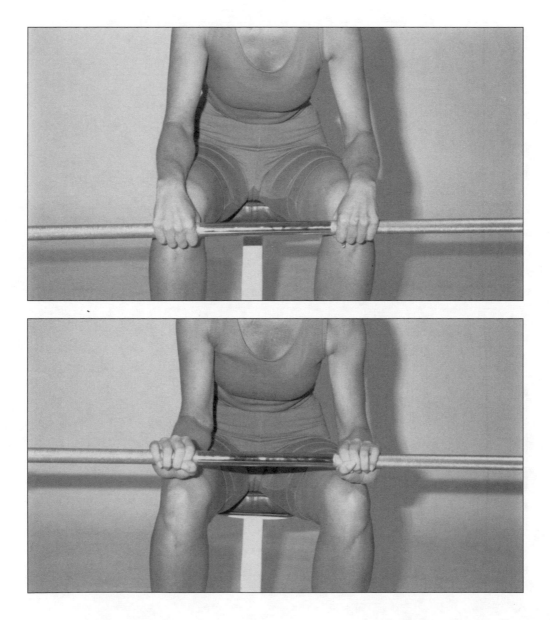

SAMPLE FREE WEIGHT WORKOUTS

Workout 1
(Largest to Smallest)

- Barbell Squat
- Stiff-Legged Dead Lift
- Dumbbell Step-Up
- Barbell Heel Raise
- Dumbbell Bent-Over Row
- Bench (Chest) Press
- Dumbbell Upright Row
- Dumbbell Triceps Extension
- Dumbbell Biceps Curl
- Abdominal Curl (p. 138)

Workout 2
(Push-Pull)

- Barbell Squat
- Barbell Heel Raise
- Dumbbell Step-Up
- Stiff-Legged Dead Lift
- Bench (Chest) Press
- Dumbbell Bent-Over Row
- Dumbbell Biceps Curl
- Dumbbell Triceps Extension
- Abdominal Curl (p. 138)

Workout 3
(Pre-Exhaustion)

- Dumbbell Step-Up
- Barbell Dead Lift
- Barbell Squat
- Barbell Heel Raise
- Dumbbell Fly
- Bench (Chest) Press
- Dumbbell Bent-Over Row
- Dumbbell Side Lateral Raise
- Abdominal Curl (p. 138)

Workout 4
(Upper Body/Lower Body)

- Bench (Chest) Press
- Barbell Squat
- Dumbbell Bent-Over Row
- Stiff-Legged Dead Lift
- Dumbbell Step-Up
- Barbell Heel Raise
- Abdominal Curl (p. 138)

CHAPTER 5

MULTISTATION EXERCISES

Multistation machines include several exercise stations as part of a single piece of equipment. These machines feature weight stacks attached to pulleys. The pulleys are connected to levers moved by the exerciser. When the levers are moved, the weight stack slides on guide rods. Because the weight stacks are on guide rods away from the exerciser, the chance of being injured by a falling weight is significantly reduced. Another positive feature of multistation machines is how easy it is to change resistance. The weight can be changed simply by removing and reinserting a metal pin. This saves you time and energy compared with free weights.

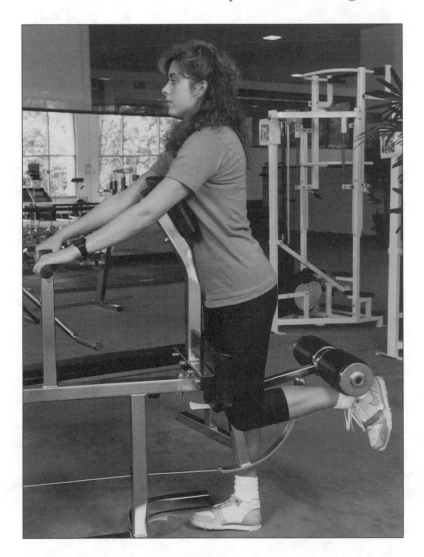

Over the years, several manufacturers have built these machines, although they have become known by the generic name *Universal Gyms*. Most of these machines are similar in appearance and design. For illustration purposes only, this chapter features exercises on machines manufactured under the name Universal Gym. If you exercise on a multistation machine sold by a different manufacturer, you should follow the manufacturer's instructions to ensure that you use it properly.

LEG PRESS

Muscles used: Gluteals, quadriceps, hamstrings.

Starting position: Sit with your shoulders against the seat back of the machine and with the balls of your feet centered on the foot pads. Adjust the seat so that your knee joints are at about a 90-degree angle. Loosely grip the handles.

Description: Straighten both of your legs, but don't lock out your knees, because this can place stress on the knee joints. Pause, then slowly recover to the starting position and repeat.

Points to emphasize:

- Don't grip the handles tightly.
- Don't allow the weight stack to bounce at the bottom of the movement.
- Don't lock out your knees at the end of the range of movement.
- Exhale during the outward press.

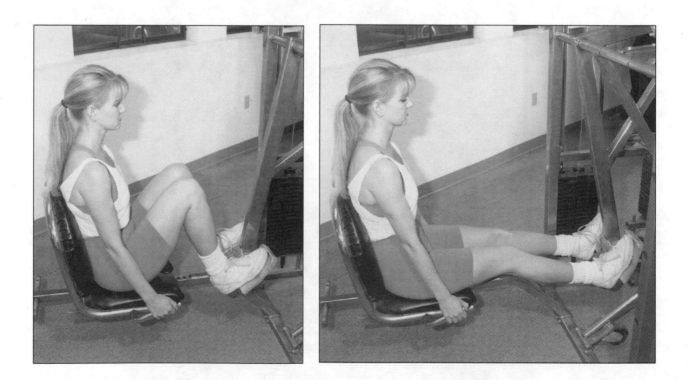

LEG EXTENSION

Muscles used: Quadriceps.

Starting position: In a seated position, put your feet behind the roller pads with the backs of your knees against the front of the seat. Keep your head and shoulders vertical.

Description: Raise your feet until both your legs are fully extended (straight). Pause, then slowly recover to the starting position and repeat.

Points to emphasize:

- Grip the sides of the bench loosely with your hands.
- Keep your hands, neck, and face muscles relaxed.

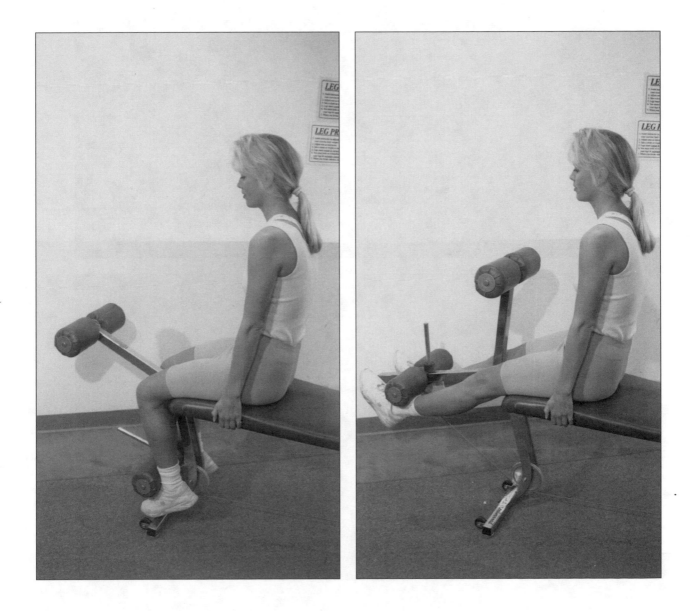

LEG CURL

Muscles used: Hamstrings.

Starting position: Lie face down on the bench. Place the backs of your ankles under the roller pads with your kneecaps just off the end of the bench.

Description: Curl your legs upward as far as possible. Pause, then slowly recover to the starting position and repeat.

Points to emphasize:

- Keep your feet in a flexed position with your toes pointing toward your knees.

- In the contracted (midrange) position of the exercise, raise your lower legs at least perpendicular to the bench (or even farther back).

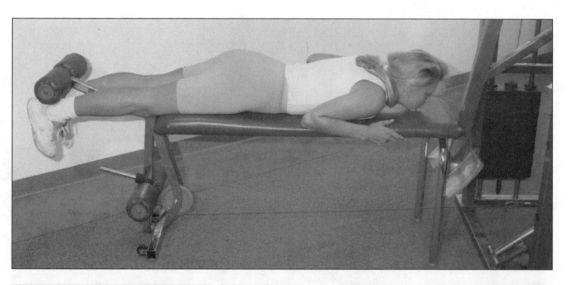

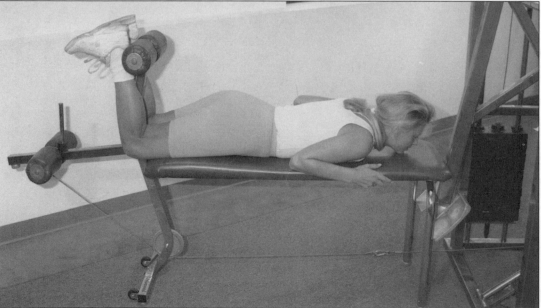

BACK EXTENSION

Muscles used: Spinal erectors, sacrospinalis.

Starting position: Firmly place your feet on the roller pad and pedal. Support your hips or stomach on the padded bar. Place your hands behind your head.

Description: From a hanging position, lift your head and trunk parallel to your hips. You can hold a weight plate behind your head to increase the resistance.

Points to emphasize:

- Don't exercise to muscular failure.
- Build the workload gradually.
- Be careful not to overwork your back in your initial workouts.
- Don't hyperextend your back in the midrange position.

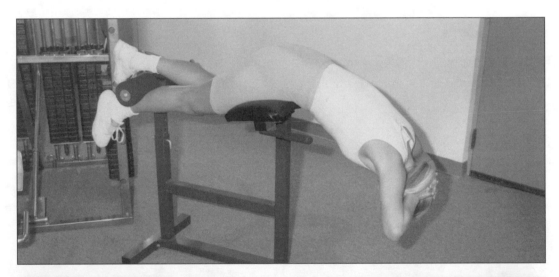

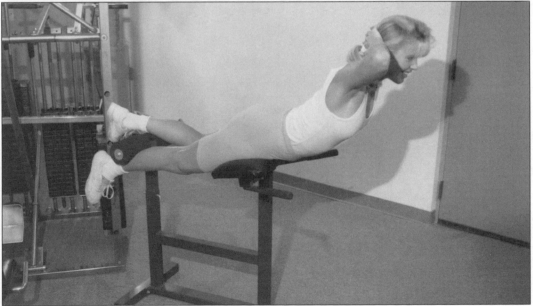

LAT PULLDOWN

Muscles used: Latissimus dorsi, biceps, rhomboids.

Starting position: Kneel facing the weight stack. Grasp the handlebar using an overhead grip slightly wider than shoulder-width.

Description: Pull the handlebar down, and touch the base of your neck. Pause, then slowly recover to the starting position and repeat.

Points to emphasize:

- Use a sitting position if preferred.
- Use an underhand grip to put more emphasis on your biceps.

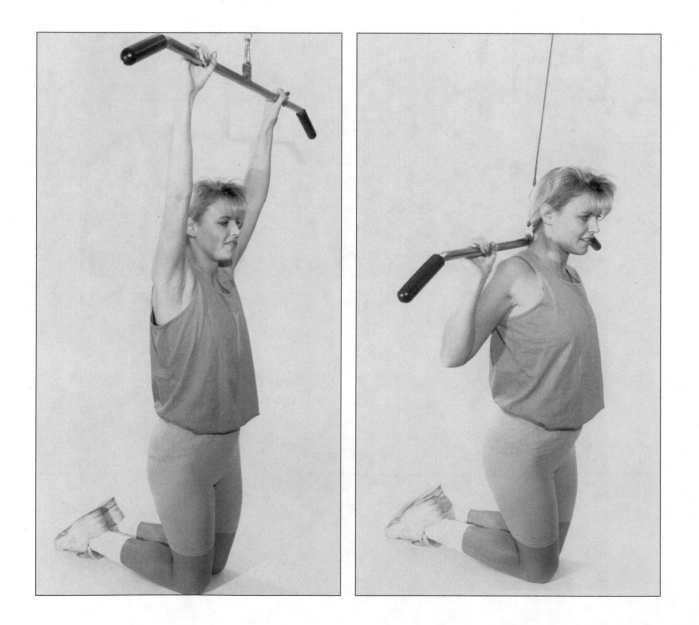

SHOULDER SHRUG

Muscles used: Trapezius.

Starting position: Stand between the chest press handles facing the weight stack. Grip the insides of the handles using an overhand grip.

Description: Keep your arms straight, and raise your shoulders as high as possible. Pause, then slowly recover to the starting position and repeat.

Points to emphasize:

- Keep your body perfectly straight.
- Allow your arms to drop as far as possible on the downward movement without bending your back.

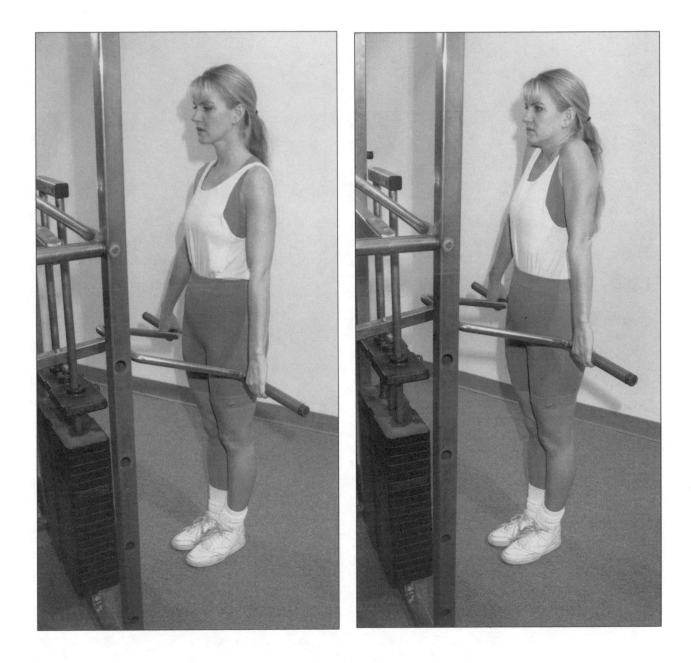

UPRIGHT ROW

Muscles used: Trapezius, deltoids, biceps.

Starting position: Stand facing the biceps curl station, and grip the handles using an overhand grip with your hands less than shoulder-width apart.

Description: Pull the bar up until it touches the underside of your chin. Pause, then slowly recover to the starting position and repeat.

Points to emphasize:

- Stand straight with your head up.
- Keep your elbows pointed to the outside.
- Pull the bar all the way to your chin.

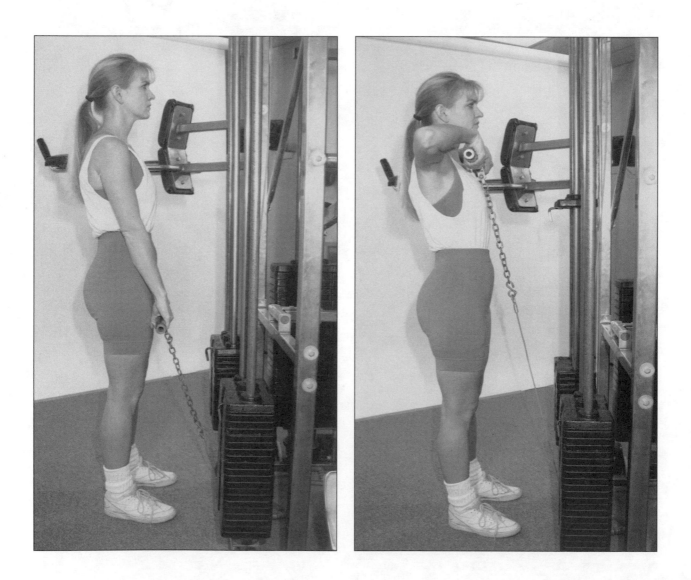

BENCH (CHEST) PRESS

Muscles used: Pectorals, deltoids, triceps.

Starting position: Lie flat on the bench with your knees bent and your feet flat touching the floor. Grip the handles using an overhand grip with your hands slightly more than shoulder-width apart.

Description: Straighten your arms until your elbows are fully extended. Pause, then slowly recover to the starting position and repeat.

Points to emphasize:

- Don't arch your back.
- Don't bounce the weight stack at the bottom.
- Exhale while raising the weight.
- You can put a block of wood under the head of the bench to increase the possible range of movement.

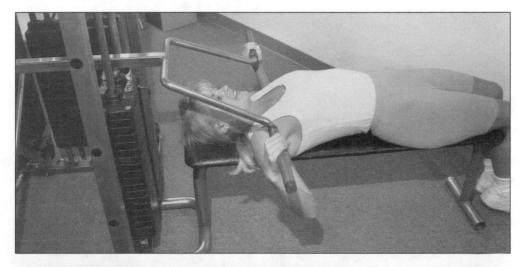

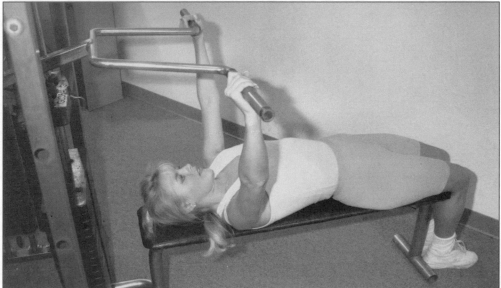

BICEPS CURL

Muscles used: Biceps.

Starting position: Stand with your arms extended downward while facing the biceps curl station. Grip the bar using an underhand grip with your hands shoulder-width apart.

Description: Curl the bar forward and upward, keeping your elbows back until the bar touches the base of your neck. Pause, then slowly recover to the starting position and repeat.

Points to emphasize:

- Don't allow your elbows to come forward.
- Keep your back straight.

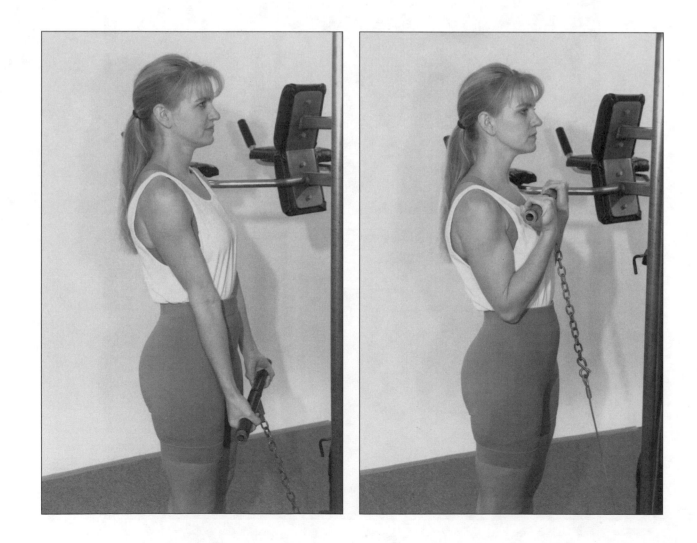

TRICEPS EXTENSION

Muscles used: Triceps.

Starting position: Stand facing the pulldown station with your feet shoulder-width apart. Grip the handlebar using an overhand grip with your hands less than shoulder-width apart. Pull the handlebar down until it is level with your shoulders.

Description: Push your hands down until your arms are extended. Pause, then slowly recover to the starting position and repeat.

Points to emphasize:

- Make sure that your elbows are always touching the sides of your body during the exercise.

- Wrap your thumbs over the bar to make it easier to stabilize your wrists.

- For greater range of movement, wrap a towel around the cable junction of the bar, grip both sides of the towel, and extend the towel downward.

- Keep your head clear of the cable.

- Control the movement when recovering to the starting position to avoid being hit with the handlebar.

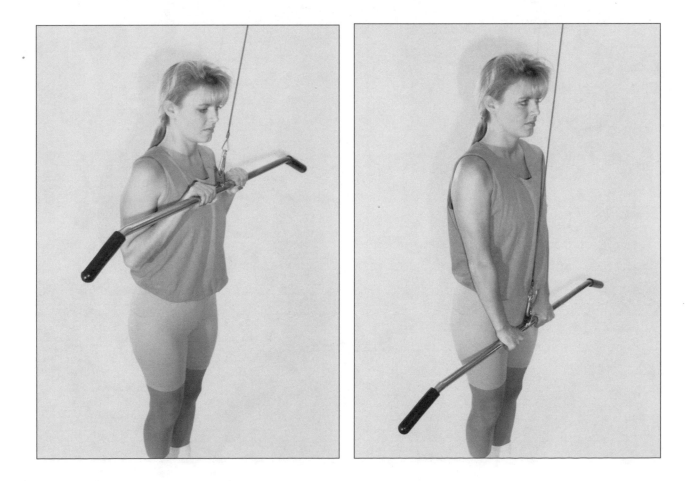

WRIST CURL

Muscles used: Forearm flexors.

Starting position: Sit on the end of an exercise bench with your forearms resting on your knees. Grasp the handles using an underhand grip, and raise the bar until the weight stack is lifted. Allow the handles to rest on your fingertips.

Description: Curl the bar up toward your elbows as far as possible. Pause, then slowly recover to the starting position and repeat.

Points to emphasize:

- Keep your forearms flat on your thighs.
- Keep your wrists just over the ends of your knees.

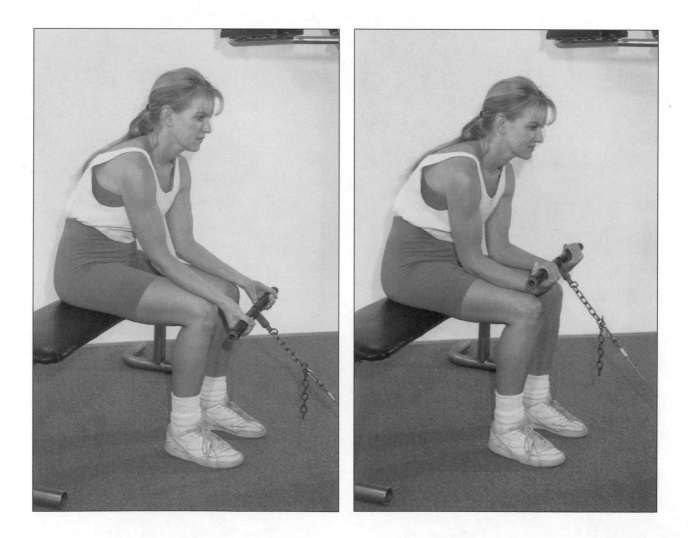

REVERSE WRIST CURL

Muscles used: Forearm extensors.

Starting position: Sit on the end of an exercise bench with your forearms resting on your knees. Grasp the handles using an overhand grip.

Description: Curl the bar up toward your elbows as far as possible. Pause, then slowly recover to the starting position and repeat.

Points to emphasize:

- Keep your forearms flat on your thighs.
- Keep your wrists just over the ends of your knees.

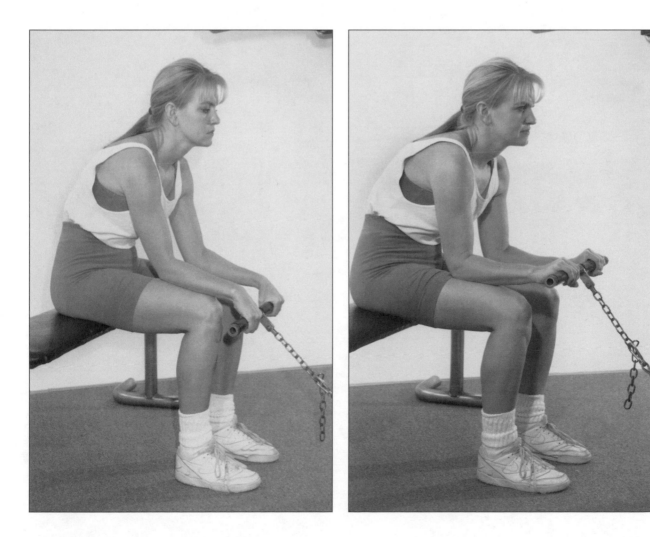

SAMPLE MULTISTATION WORKOUTS

Workout 1
(Largest to Smallest)

- Leg Press
- Back Extension
- Leg Extension
- Leg Curl
- Lat Pulldown
- Bench (Chest) Press
- Upright Row
- Triceps Extension
- Biceps Curl
- Abdominal Curl (p. 138)

Workout 2
(Push-Pull)

- Leg Press
- Leg Curl
- Leg Extension
- Bench (Chest) Press
- Lat Pulldown
- Biceps Curl
- Triceps Extension
- Abdominal Curl (p. 138)

Workout 3
(Pre-Exhaustion)

- Leg Curl
- Leg Extension
- Leg Press
- Triceps Extension
- Bench (Chest) Press
- Biceps Curl
- Lat Pulldown
- Back Extension
- Abdominal Curl (p. 138)

Workout 4
(Upper Body/Lower Body)

- Bench (Chest) Press
- Leg Press
- Lat Pulldown
- Leg Extension
- Leg Curl
- Abdominal Curl (p. 138)

CHAPTER 6

VARIABLE RESISTANCE EXERCISES

Variable resistance machines include equipment that varies the force (resistance) the exerciser must overcome through the exercise range of motion. As previously discussed, your muscles aren't equally strong throughout their full range of movement. In any free weight exercise and most multistation machine exercises, a "sticking" point exists. Once you're past this point, continued movement of the weight is easier. Thus, free weight and most multistation machines are limited to the maximum resistance that can be handled at the sticking point in an exercise. Variable resistance machines use a cam or other mechanical device to vary the resistance and match the leverage advantages and disadvantages that occur over the range of any exercise movement.

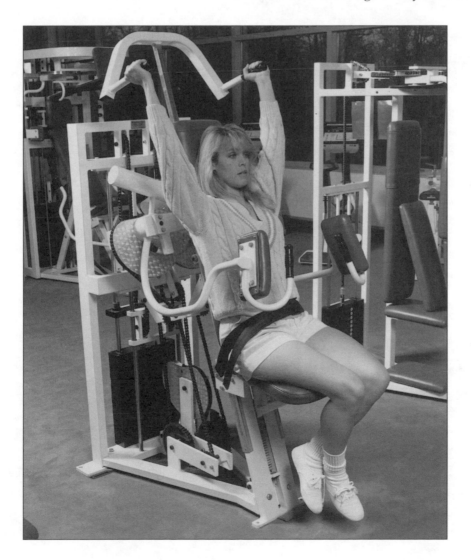

For illustration purposes only, this chapter features exercises on Nautilus machines. If you exercise on a different type of equipment, you should follow the manufacturer's instructions to ensure that you use it properly. Note that different manufacturers vary the names assigned to each machine.

BACK EXTENSION

Muscles used: Gluteus maximus, spinal erectors.

Starting position: Sit down on the machine with your lower and upper back against the rear support pads. Fasten the seat belts snugly around your thighs. Tuck your chin and cross your arms over your chest.

Description: From the starting position, push back through approximately a 60-degree range of motion.

Points to emphasize:

- To avoid injury, perform the back extension in a slow, controlled manner.
- Be careful not to arch your back excessively.

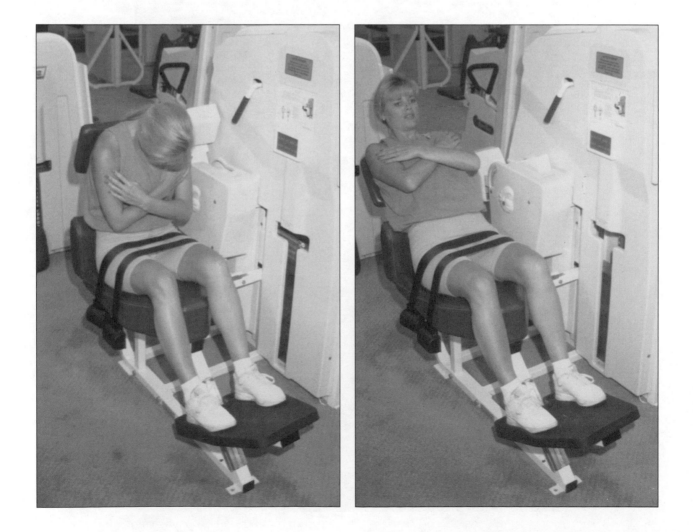

LEG PRESS

Muscles used: Gluteus maximus, quadriceps, hamstrings.

Starting position: Sit down on the leg press machine so that your back is flush against the support pad. Place your feet on the pads with your toes turned slightly inward and your knees bent at a 90-degree angle.

Description: Push both of your legs outward until your knees are almost straight. Pause with your knees slightly bent, then slowly recover to the starting position and repeat.

Points to emphasize:

- Relax your hands, neck, and face muscles.
- Always keep your head, back, and buttocks against the support pads.
- Avoid locking your knees out when your legs are in the extended position.

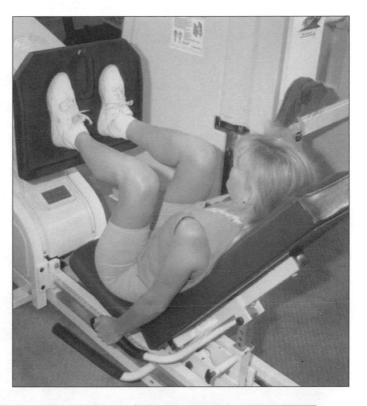

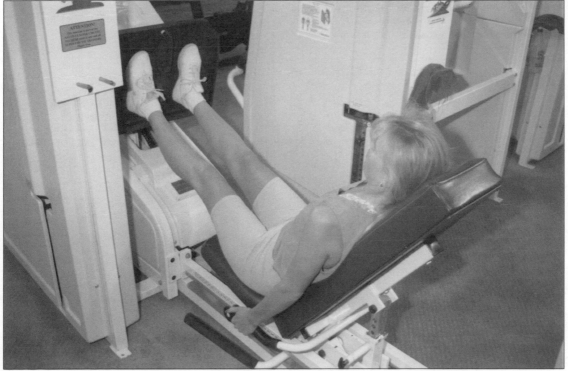

LEG EXTENSION

Muscles used: Quadriceps.

Starting position: In a seated position, place both feet behind the roller pads with the backs of your knees against the front of the seat. Adjust the seat back so it touches your lower back.

Description: Raise your feet until both of your legs are straight. Pause, then recover to the starting position and repeat. Keep your head and shoulders against the seat back.

Points to emphasize:

- Pause when you reach the fully contracted position.
- Keep your hand, neck, and face muscles relaxed.

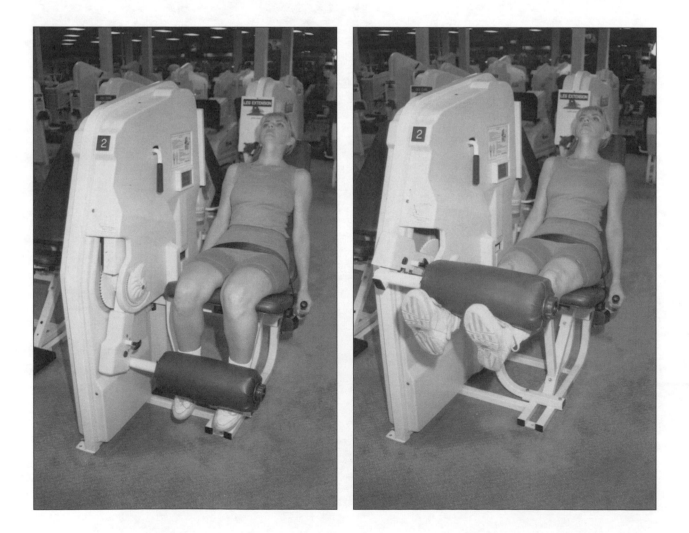

LEG CURL

Muscles used: Hamstrings.

Starting position: Lie face down on the machine. Place the backs of your ankles under the roller pads with your kneecaps just off the end of the bench. Grip the handles loosely.

Description: Curl your legs upward, attempting to touch your buttocks with the roller pads. Pause, then slowly recover to the starting position.

Points to emphasize:

- Keep your feet flexed.
- Allow your hips to rise off the bench when nearing full contraction.

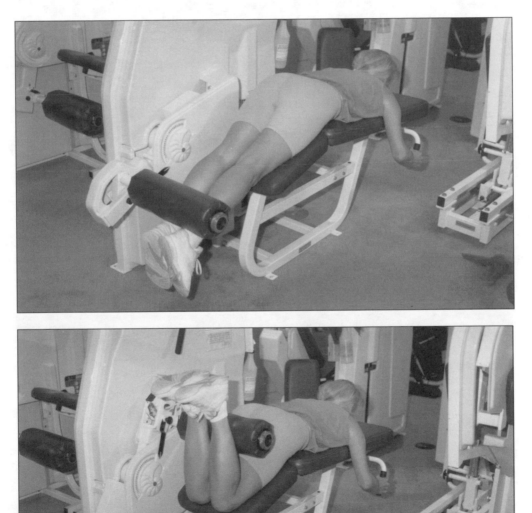

HIP ABDUCTION

Muscles used: Gluteus medius, gluteus minimus, quadriceps.

Starting position: Sit on the machine, and place your knees and calves on the movement arms. Your outer thighs and knees should be firmly against the resistance pads. Keep your head and shoulders relaxed against the seat back.

Description: Spread your knees and thighs to the widest possible position. Pause, then recover slowly to the starting position and repeat.

Point to emphasize:

- Keep your head and shoulders against the support pad.

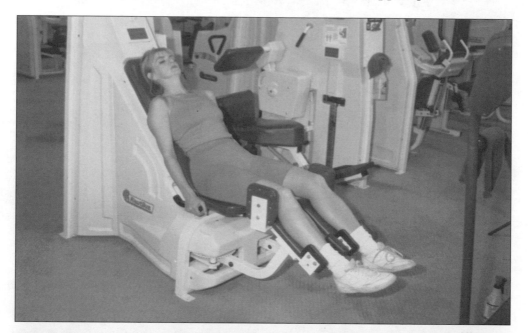

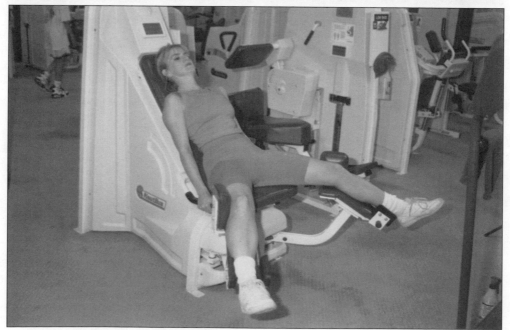

HIP ADDUCTION

Muscles used: Adductor magnus.

Starting position: Move the thigh pads to the inside position. Sit in the machine, and place your knees and calves on the movement arms. Your inner thighs and knees should be firmly against the resistance pads. Keep your head and shoulders relaxed against the seat back.

Description: Press (pull) your knees and thighs smoothly together. Pause, then return slowly to the starting position and repeat.

Point to emphasize:

- Keep your head and shoulders against the support pad.

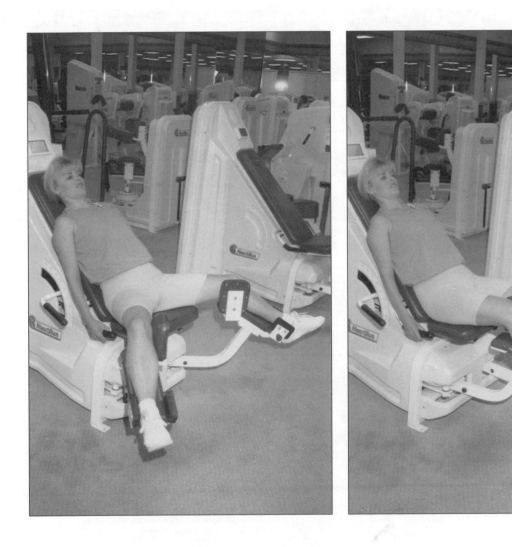

HEEL RAISE

Muscles used: Calves.

Starting position: Adjust the belt comfortably around your hips. Stand on the balls of your feet on the first step, while placing your hands on the dip bars and keeping your back erect.

Description: Raise your heels as high as possible. Pause, then slowly recover to the starting position and repeat. Keep your knees locked.

Points to emphasize:

- Don't lean forward.
- Flex your toes upward at the bottom of the movement to allow for a maximum stretch.

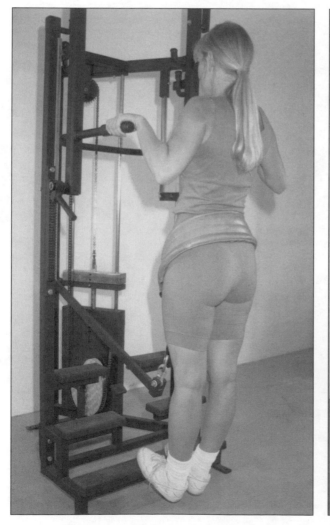 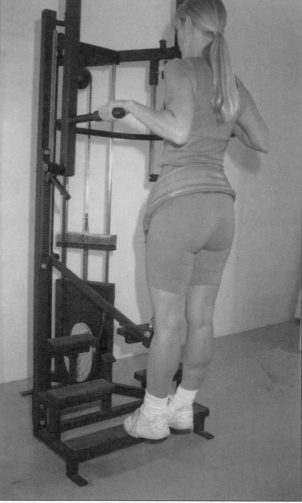

ARM CROSS

Muscles used: Pectoralis major, deltoids.

Starting position: Lie down with your back flat on the bench and your feet on the footrest. Place your arms around the roller pads with your palms facing forward.

Description: Keeping your head, shoulders, and back firmly pressed against the bench, move your arms together until the roller pads touch. Pause, then slowly recover to the starting position and repeat.

Points to emphasize:

- Keep your palms facing forward.
- Keep your head, shoulders, and back firmly pressed against the bench.

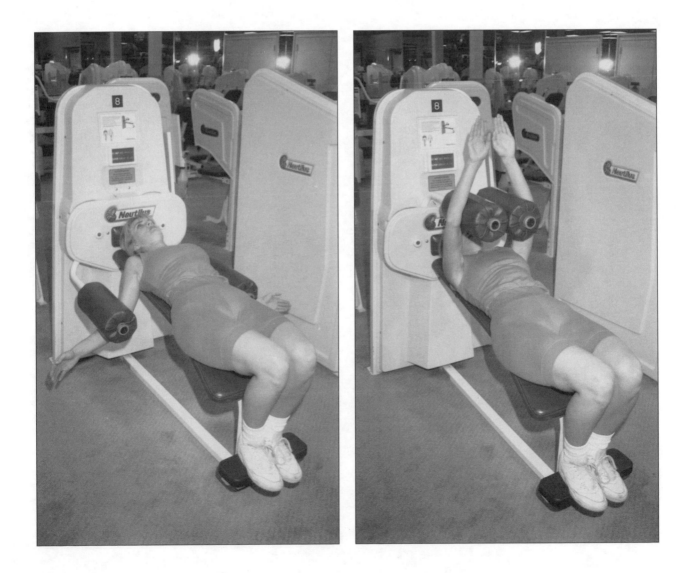

SEATED ROW

Muscles used: Latissimus dorsi, rhomboids, biceps, and posterior deltoids.

Starting position: Adjust your seat to the proper height, sit with your chest against the support pad, and grasp the handlebars.

Description: Pull the handlebars toward your chest. Pause, then slowly recover to the starting position and repeat.

Points to emphasize:

- Keep your chest against the support.
- Pull the handlebars back as far as possible.

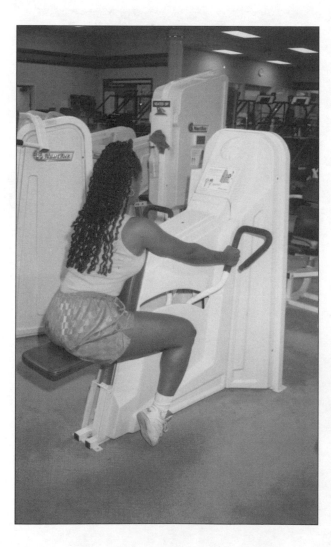
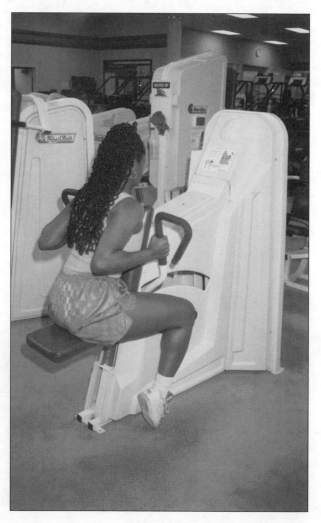

SEATED PRESS

Muscles used: Deltoids, triceps, trapezius.

Starting position: Sit with your hands grasping the seated press handles; rest your back against the support pad.

Description: Extend your arms fully upward. Pause, then recover to the starting position and repeat.

Points to emphasize:

- Do not arch your back—keep it firmly pressed against the support pad.

- Do not rest in the "locked-out" (midrange) position.

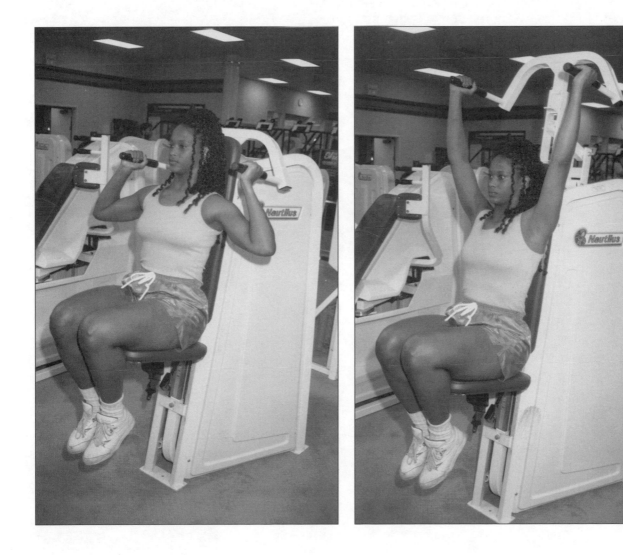

PULLOVER

Muscles used: Latissimus dorsi.

Starting position: Adjust the seat so that the center of each shoulder joint is aligned with the center of the cam. Fasten the seat belt tightly. Depress the foot pedals to move the elbow pads forward. Place the backs of your elbows on the pads. Your hands should be open and leaning against the groove in the curved portion of the bar. Remove your feet from the foot pedals, and allow your elbows to move back slowly to a stretched starting position.

Description: Rotate your elbows forward and downward until the crossbar touches your hips. Pause, then slowly recover to the starting position and repeat. To reduce the stress on your lower back, your head and shoulders should curl forward during the exercise.

Points to emphasize:

- Keep your head and shoulders against the back of the seat.
- Keep your hands open and relaxed.
- Allow your elbows to stretch back as far as possible at the completion of each repetition.

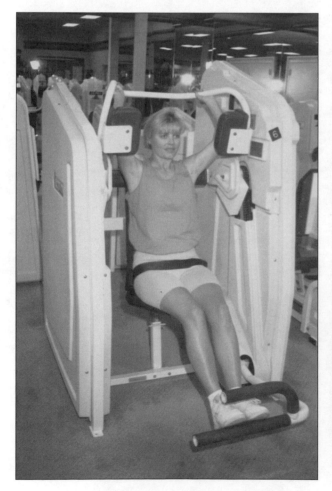
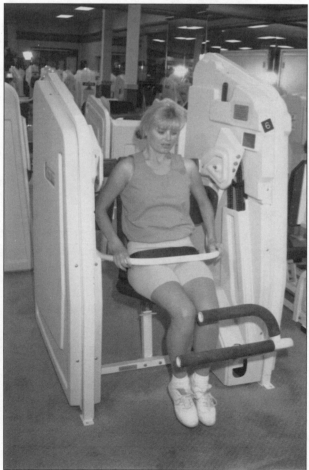

SIDE LATERAL RAISE

Muscles used: Deltoids (medial).

Starting position: Sit with your shoulders aligned with the axis of rotation of the cam. Place your upper arms against the arm support pads and grasp the hand grips. Your back, head, and shoulders rest against the rear support pad.

Description: Leading with your elbows, raise your arms upward until your forearms are parallel to the floor. Pause, then slowly recover to the starting position and repeat.

Points to emphasize:

- Lead with your elbows and not with your hands.
- Keep your head, back, and shoulder blades firmly pressed against the rear support pad.

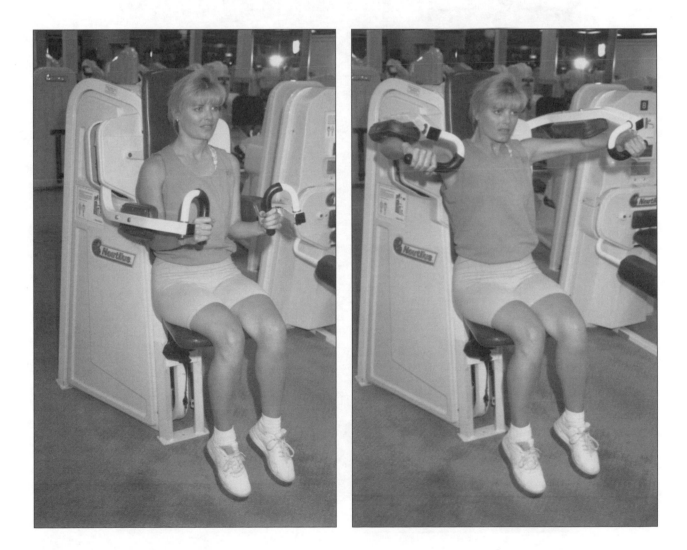

BICEPS CURL

Muscles used: Biceps.

Starting position: In a seated position, place your elbows on the pad and align them with the center of the cams. Adjust the seat so that your shoulders are slightly lower than your elbows.

Description: Curl both of your arms to a point where your lower arms are slightly past 90 degrees. Pause, then slowly recover to the starting position and repeat.

Points to emphasize:

- Keep your wrists locked.
- Don't allow your elbows to come off the pads.
- Keep your head and torso erect.

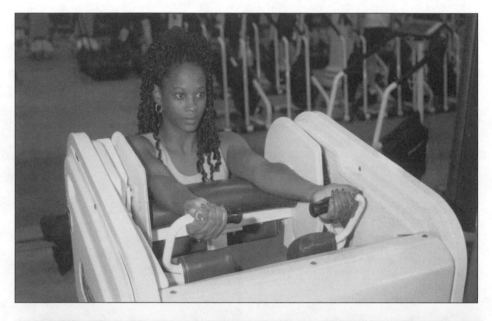

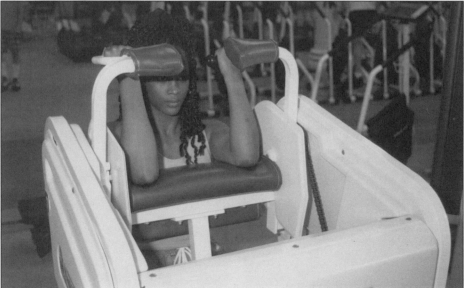

SEATED DIP

Muscles used: Triceps, pectorals, deltoids.

Starting position: Adjust the seat height so that when you are seated and you grasp the handles, a 90-degree or less angle is formed at your elbow joint. Grasp the handles with an overhand grip and keep your back, head, and shoulder blades against the rear support pad.

Description: Press the handles down until your arms are fully extended. Pause, then slowly recover to the starting position and repeat.

Points to emphasize:

- Concentrate on elbow extension.
- Keep your head, back, and shoulder blades firmly pressed against the rear support pad.

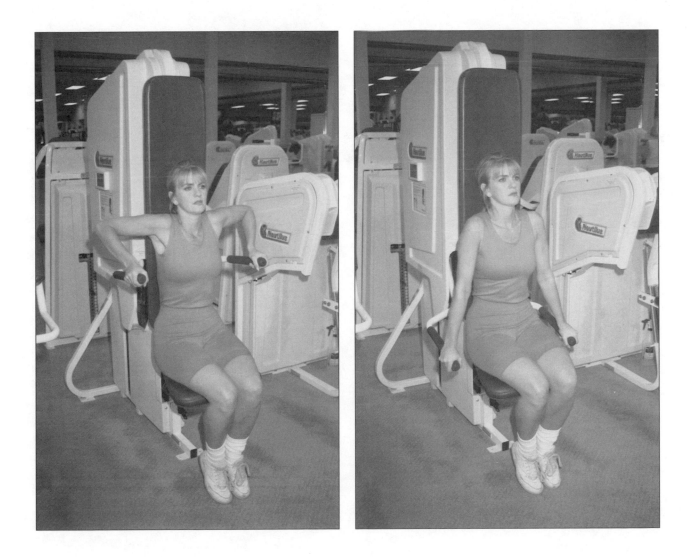

ABDOMINAL CURL

Muscles used: Adbominals.

Starting position: Adjust the seat so that your elbows fit comfortably on the arm support pad. Fasten the seat belt snugly around your thighs and grasp the hand grips while placing your elbows on the support pads.

Description: Curl your trunk approximately 60° forward. Pause, then slowly recover to the starting position and repeat.

Point to emphasize:

• Avoid pulling down with your hands and arms.

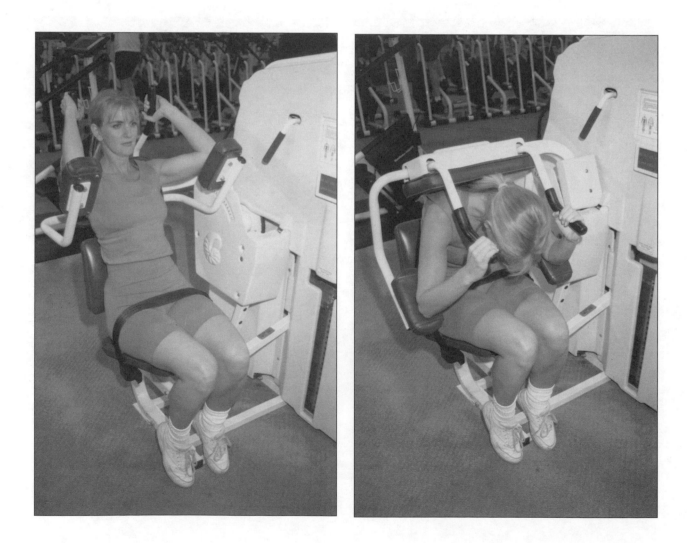

Sample Variable Resistance Workouts

Workout 1
(Largest to Smallest)

- Leg Press
- Back Extension
- Leg Extension
- Leg Curl
- Heel Raise
- Pullover
- Arm Cross
- Seated Press
- Seated Dip
- Biceps Curl
- Abdominal Curl

Workout 2
(Push-Pull)

- Leg Press
- Leg Curl
- Leg Extension
- Heel Raise
- Back Extension
- Arm Cross
- Pullover
- Seated Press
- Biceps Curl
- Seated Dip
- Abdominal Curl

Workout 3
(Pre-Exhaustion)

- Leg Extension
- Leg Press
- Leg Curl
- Back Extension
- Arm Cross
- Seated Dip
- Pullover
- Seated Row
- Side Lateral Raise
- Seated Press
- Abdominal Curl

Workout 4
(Upper Body/Lower Body)

- Arm Cross
- Leg Extension
- Pullover
- Leg Curl
- Seated Press
- Hip Abduction
- Seated Row
- Hip Adduction
- Seated Dip
- Heel Raise
- Abdominal Curl

CHAPTER 7

STRENGTH TRAINING WITHOUT EQUIPMENT

As we've discussed, to develop muscle strength and endurance, you only have to take one step—put a demand on the muscle or muscle group you want to improve. Apply resistance to a muscle that is greater than the muscle is used to handling (placing an overload on your muscles).

The *type* of resistance is not the key to improving muscle strength. Your muscles have neither eyes nor brains. They don't know if you're using rocks, free weights, or sandbags as the source of resistance. Regardless of the type of resistance you use, the critical factors influencing your improvement are how well you apply the resistance and what load you put on the muscle.

Positive alternatives exist for developing muscle strength that don't require much (if any) equipment. Three of the most effective techniques using little or no equipment are negative-only, buddy, and stick exercises.

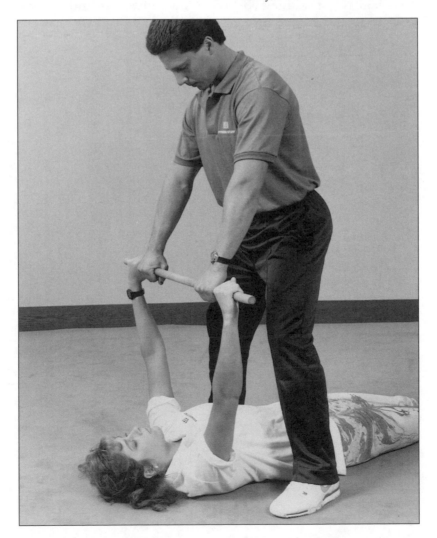

NEGATIVE-ONLY EXERCISES

Negative-only exercises are based on the principle that the muscles you use to raise a weight are the same muscles you use to lower (under control) that weight. When you lift a weight, your muscles are shortening. This part of an exercise is the concentric or positive phase. When you lower a weight, your muscles are lengthening—the eccentric or negative phase of the lift. Negative-only exercises are calisthenic exercises that involve doing only the negative phase of the exercise.

NEGATIVE-ONLY PUSH-UPS

Muscles used: Deltoids, pectorals, triceps.

Starting position: From an all-fours position, extend and lock your knees to assume a front leaning rest position. Keep your back straight.

Description: With your body supported on your fully extended arms and toes, slowly lower your body to the floor by bending your elbows. The lowering (negative-only) movement should take 3 to 4 seconds. Once your body touches the floor, you should relax, reassume an all-fours position, and recover to the starting position. Repeat the exercise.

Point to emphasize:

- A partner can add resistance beyond the weight of your body by straddling you as you do the exercise and applying a limited downward force to the middle of your back.

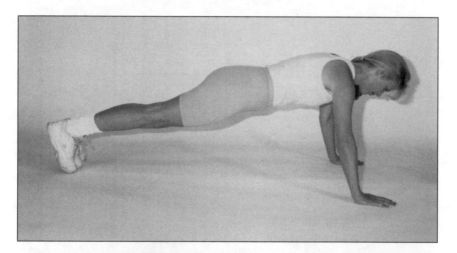

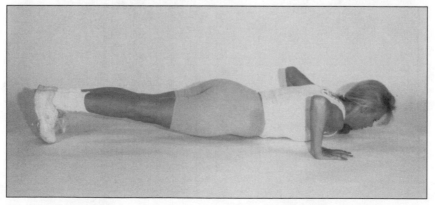

NEGATIVE-ONLY CHIN-UPS

Muscles used: Latissimus dorsi, biceps.

Starting position: Hang from a chinning bar in a flexed-arm position with your chin over the bar; use an underhand grip, with your hands slightly closer than shoulder-width apart and your elbows pulled back. If necessary, bend your legs to keep them from touching the floor.

Description: Slowly lower yourself to the fully extended position. The movement through the eccentric (negative) phase should take at least 3 to 4 seconds. Drop off, and then remount the bar using steps. Pause, then repeat the exercise.

Points to emphasize:

- Don't grip the bar too tightly.
- This exercise can also be performed using an overhand grip (pull-up).
- Pause momentarily before beginning the lowering phase of the exercise.
- Use steps high enough (e.g., a ladder) so you don't have to jump to get your chin over the bar.
- Either a weight belt or a partner pulling downward on your hips can provide additional resistance.

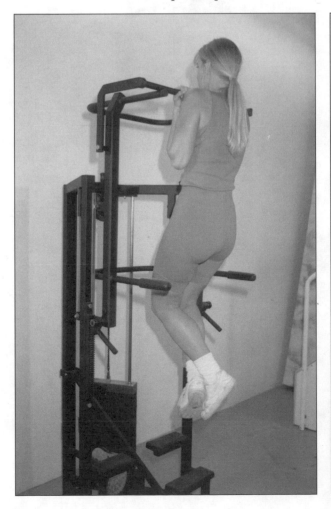 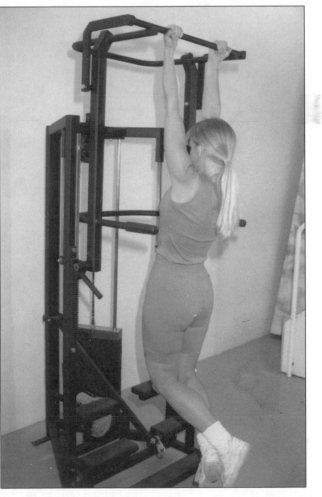

NEGATIVE-ONLY DIPS

Muscles used: Triceps, pectorals, deltoids.

Starting position: Use steps (e.g., a ladder, a stool, or a box) to mount the dip bars. With your arms extended, grip the bars with your hands facing inward; suspend your weight on your hands. Keep your knees slightly bent so that your feet don't touch the floor.

Description: Slowly lower your body as far as possible, taking about 3 to 4 seconds. Relax, and then recover to the starting position using the steps again. Pause, then repeat the exercise.

Points to emphasize:

- Don't let your feet touch the floor before you have slowly lowered yourself through a full range of movement.

- You can wear a weighted belt or have a partner put a downward force on your hips as you lower yourself if you want more resistance.

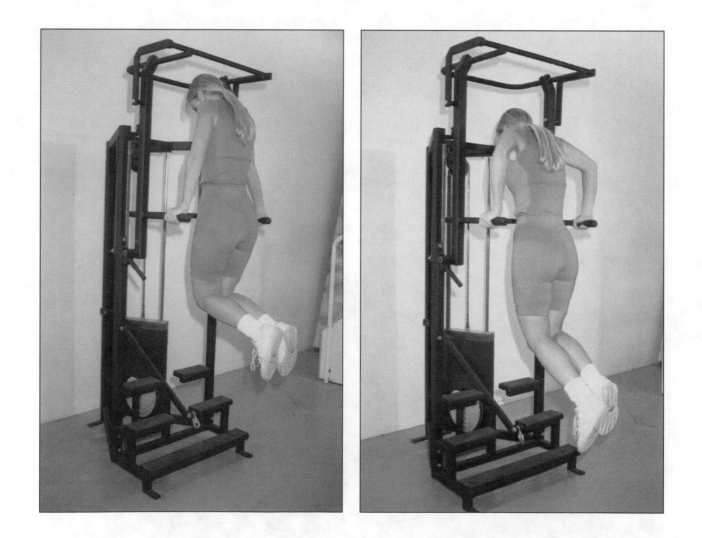

NEGATIVE-ONLY SIT-UPS

Muscles used: Abdominals, hip flexors, quadriceps.

Starting position: Sit with your feet together and secured, either by a partner or underneath a heavy object. Your knees should be bent and together; your hands should be either interlocked behind your head or held close to your chest.

Description: Slowly lower your back to the floor, taking 3 to 4 seconds. Always keep your buttocks in contact with the floor. When your back touches the floor, relax, and use your hands to get back to the starting position. Pause, then repeat the exercise.

Points to emphasize:

- In the starting position, keep your body perpendicular to the floor.

- Additional resistance can be provided by holding an object (e.g., a barbell plate) close to your chest.

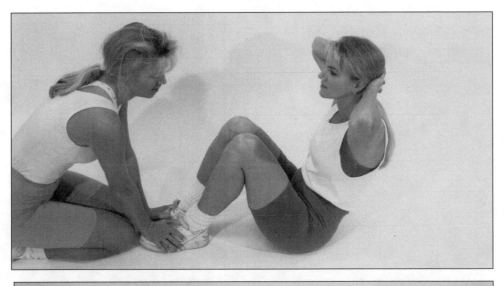

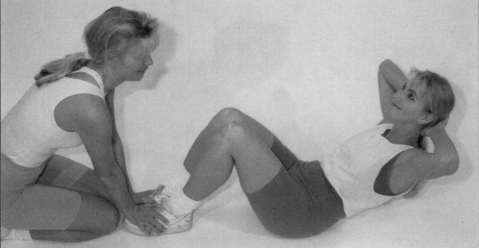

Buddy Exercises

Buddy exercises are done with the exerciser moving against force exerted by a buddy (partner). Also called manual resistance exercises and partner resistance exercises (PREs), buddy exercises have been used since the early 20th century to develop strength. In recent years, buddy exercises have been used by the military and many athletic teams to develop muscular fitness. Buddy exercises can be used to develop any major muscle group in your body.

LEG PRESS

Muscles used: Gluteus maximus, quadriceps, hamstrings, spinal erectors.

Starting position: Lie on your back with one or both feet on the spotter's chest. Use a pad between you and your partner to put your feet on during the exercise. Extend your arms for balance. Your training partner's body weight serves as the resistance.

Description: Extend one or both legs slowly. Pause, and recover to the starting position. Repeat the exercise. Don't lock your knees out in the midrange position of the exercise.

Point to emphasize:

• This exercise can be done one leg at a time or both legs together.

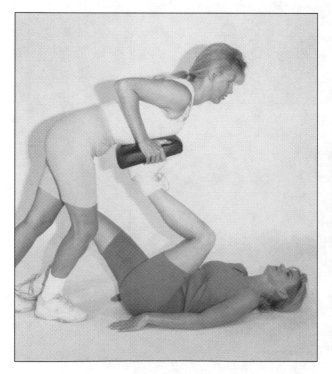 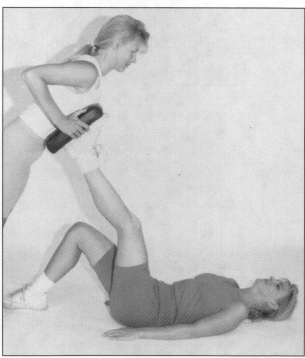

LEG CURL

Muscles used: Hamstrings.

Starting position: Lie face down. Flex your toes to increase the effective range of motion for your hamstrings. The resistance should be applied to the backside of your heel or leg. If necessary, your partner should use both hands to spot.

Description: While raising your leg, flex your toes toward your knee. Keep your foot in this position until your toes almost touch the ground. Raise your lower leg as high as possible, and pause before recovering to the starting position. Repeat the exercise.

Point to emphasize:

- Do this exercise with one leg for a specific number of repetitions before switching to the other leg.

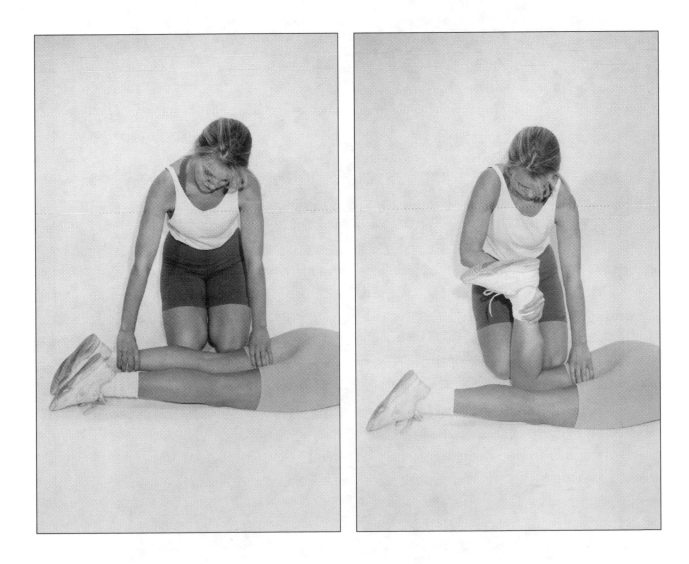

HIP ABDUCTION

Muscles used: Gluteus medius, gluteus minimus.

Starting position: Lie on your side with your body extended. Your legs should be slightly separated. Your upper and lower body remain perfectly aligned. Don't allow your upper body to bend forward at the waist. Your training partner applies resistance to the side of your leg. If you have a history of knee problems, the resistance should be applied just above your knee.

Description: Raise your leg sideward and upward as high as possible. Pause in the contracted position before recovering to the starting position. Repeat the exercise.

Point to emphasize:

- Do the exercise with one leg for a specific number of repetitions before switching to the other leg.

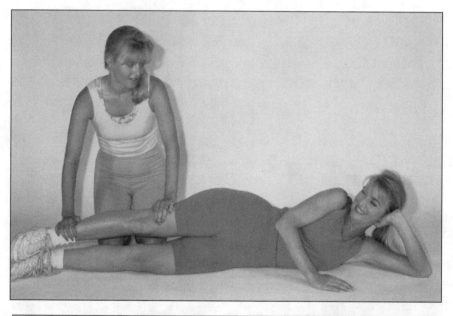

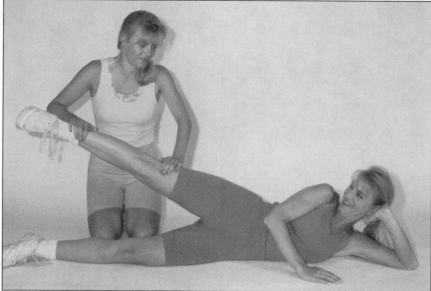

HIP ADDUCTION

Muscles used: Adductor magnus.

Starting position: Sit with your legs bent and feet pressed together. Your partner applies resistance to the inside of your knees. The spotter should be careful as you approach the fully stretched position (i.e., when your legs are apart). An injury is possible if the spotter applies too much resistance while you're in the stretched position.

Description: Pull your knees toward each other, against the resistance, until they reach the contracted position (i.e., they're touching each other). Pause and recover to the starting position. Repeat the exercise.

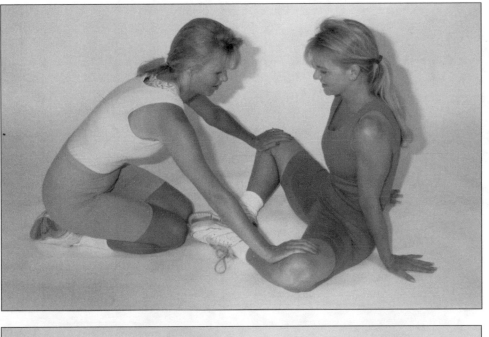

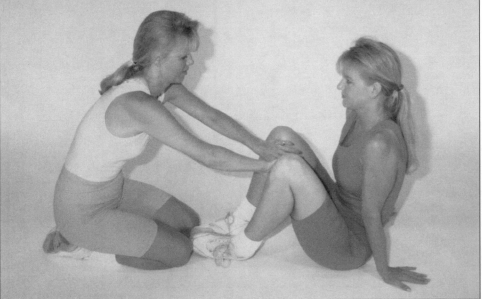

HIP FLEXION

Muscles used: Hip flexors.

Starting position: Lie on your back. The resistance should be applied just above your knee. The spotter must move backward and forward as you raise and lower your leg.

Description: Flex your hip, raising your knee toward your chest. Pause in the contracted position before recovering to the starting position. Repeat the exercise.

Point to emphasize:

• This exercise can be done with one leg at a time or both legs together.

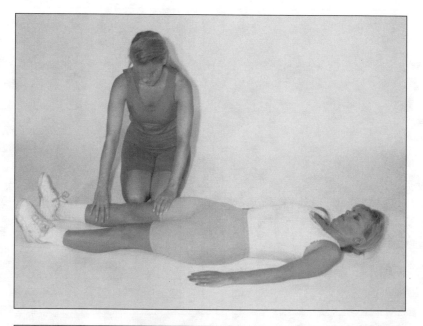

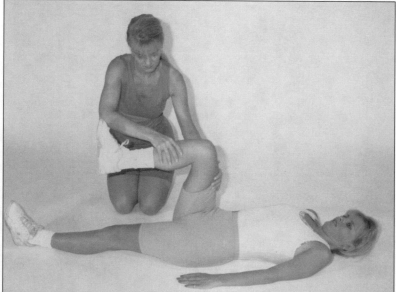

HEEL RAISE

Muscles used: Calves.

Starting position: Sit on a flat bench with the balls of your feet on a wooden block—this will allow you to obtain a stretch in the starting position. Your training partner can provide resistance by sitting on top of your thighs just above your knees. The exercise can also be done one leg at a time, with or without a spotter.

Description: Elevate your heels as high as possible, and pause before recovering to the starting position. Repeat the exercise.

Points to emphasize:

- Raise your heels as high as possible for each repetition.
- Start with your heels as low as possible.
- Keep your back straight.

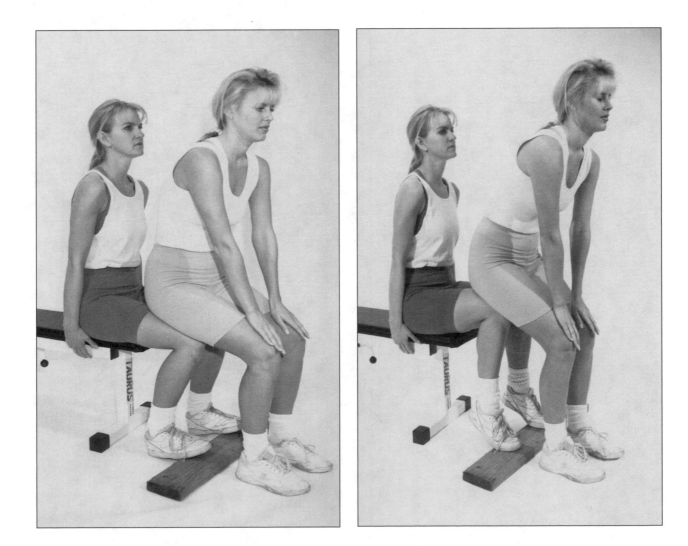

FRONT RAISE

Muscles used: Anterior deltoid, pectorals.

Starting position: Stand and then stagger your feet about half of a walking step apart for balance. Your body should stay erect. Extend your arms rearward from your body with your palms facing away. Keep your arms shoulder-width apart.

Description: Raise your arms forward and upward to a position overhead, and pause before recovering to the starting position. The resistance should be applied to the top of your wrists and hands. The spotter must move backward and forward during the raising and lowering of your arms so your arms can remain extended.

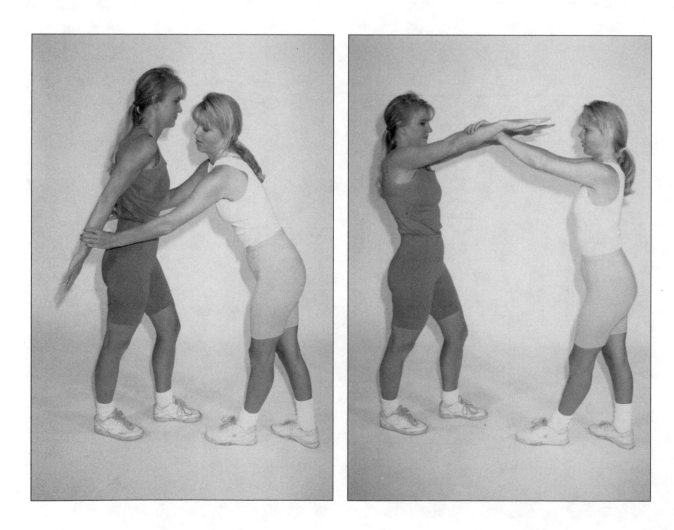

BENT-ARM FLY

Muscles used: Pectorals, anterior deltoid, subscapularis.

Starting position: Lie on your back with your arms bent at 90° and your upper arm perpendicular to your body.

Description: Raise your elbow(s) upward and toward the midline of your body. Pause, then recover to the starting position. The resistance should be applied to the inside of your arm(s). Repeat the exercise. The exercise is easier to spot one arm at a time but can be done with both arms.

Point to emphasize:

- Because the muscles being exercised are stronger than the muscles being used to spot, allow less time (2 seconds) for the lowering phase if both of your arms are exercised together.

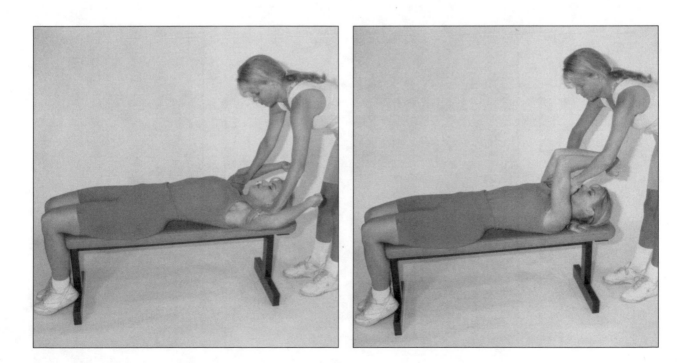

INTERNAL ROTATION

Muscles used: Subscapularis.

Starting position: Lie on your back with your elbow bent at 90°
and your upper arm perpendicular to your body. The palm
of your hand should be facing skyward with your arm in a
comfortable position. Don't put your shoulder in a
hyperstretched position.

Description: Contract your rotators completely by moving your
arm through a full range of motion around a vertical plane
to your body. Pause before recovering to the starting position. The resistance should be applied to your wrist and to
the palm of your hand. Be careful that you don't overexert.
For your first several workouts, don't give a maximal exertion. Change arms and repeat the exercise.

Point to emphasize:

- The range of motion of the subscapularis muscle varies from
  person to person.

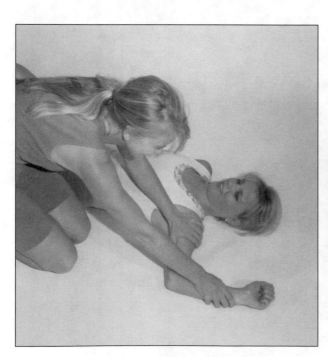 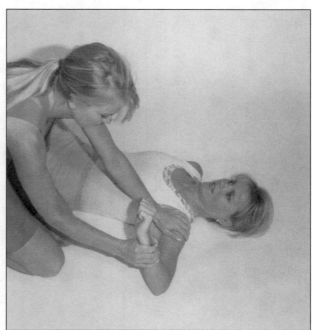

EXTERNAL ROTATION

Muscles used: Rotator cuff muscles (infraspinatus and teres minor).

Starting position: Use the same starting position as for the internal rotation exercise, except for the position of your arm. Your arm should be in a forward position with your palm facing the ground.

Description: Move your arm up toward the spotter through a full range of motion. Keep your upper arm in contact with the floor. The resistance should be applied to the back of your hand and wrist. Change arms and repeat the exercise.

Point to emphasize:

- Use less than maximum effort during your first several workouts to avoid overexerting these underdeveloped muscles.

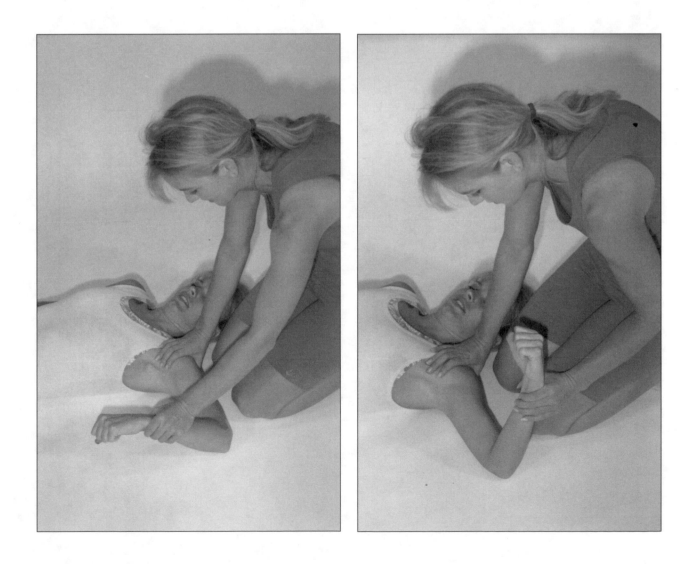

BENT-OVER SIDE LATERAL RAISE

Muscles used: Posterior deltoid, rhomboids, trapezius.

Starting position: Your upper body should be bent at the waist and parallel to the ground, with your arms extended and hanging downward. Your arms should be crossed to provide maximum stretching. Don't bend your arms.

Description: Raise your arms sideward and upward to a position where they are parallel to the floor and perpendicular to your upper body. Pause in the contracted position, then recover to the starting position. Repeat the exercise. The resistance should be applied to the backside of your wrists or elbows.

Points to emphasize:

* Keep your head up and your back straight.
* Keep your back parallel to the floor.

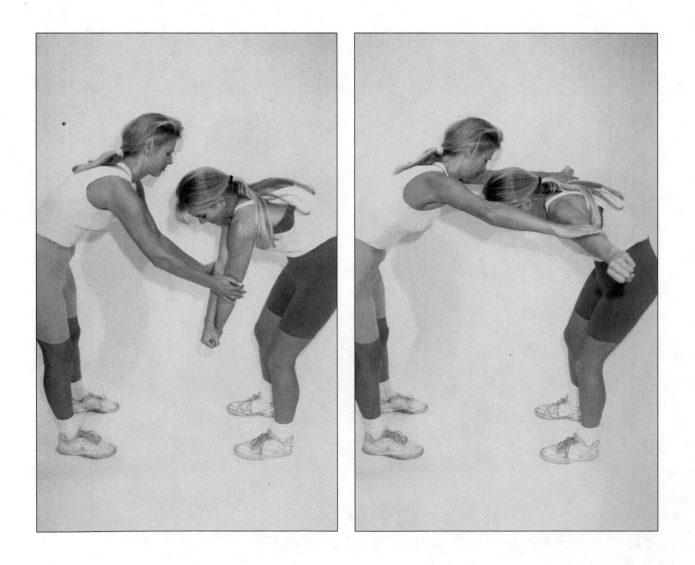

STICK EXERCISES

Stick exercises are buddy exercises designed to develop your upper body muscles. They use a wooden dowel or other cylindrical device (a broomstick, a baseball bat, a rifle, etc.). Although buddy exercises not using a stick do exist for the upper body, the wooden dowel gives an added degree of comfort and control. The conditioning program at the United States Military Academy uses a 30-in. wooden dowel to perform stick exercises. At the minimum, the dowel should be as long as the width of the exerciser's shoulders. Stick exercises usually combine two movements into one exercise.

BACK PULLDOWN/BENCH (CHEST) PRESS

Muscles used: Rhomboids, pectorals, deltoids, triceps, biceps.

Starting position: Lie on a flat bench and thrust your arms overhead, shoulder-width apart, palms up. Your partner should straddle your chest, facing toward your arms and head. A bar or wooden dowel should be put in your hands by your partner.

Description: Pull the bar toward your chest against resistance provided by your partner. Pause, then push (press) the bar back to the starting position against the resistance of your partner. Repeat the exercise.

Point to emphasize:

- Both movements (the pulldown and the press) should be done slowly, taking 3 to 4 seconds for each direction.

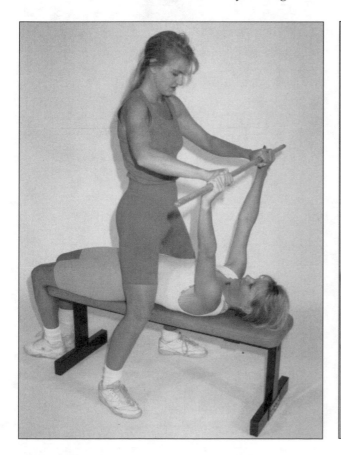
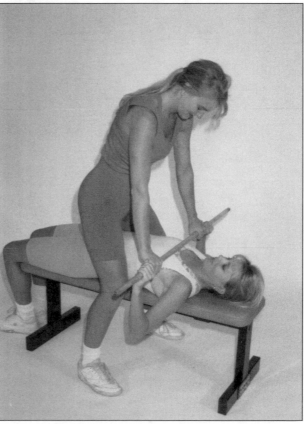

LAT PULLDOWN/SHOULDER PRESS

Muscles used: Latissimus dorsi, biceps, deltoids, triceps.

Starting position: Sit with your legs crossed. Raise your arms overhead with your palms up. Your partner stands behind you and places a knee in the middle of your back to give you stability. A bar or wooden dowel should be put in your hands by your partner.

Description: Pull the bar straight down, and touch the base of your neck. Your partner provides resistance against your movement. Pause, then push (press) the bar back to the starting position against the resistance of your partner. Repeat the exercise.

Point to emphasize:

- Both movements (the pulldown and the press) should be done slowly, taking 3 to 4 seconds for each direction.

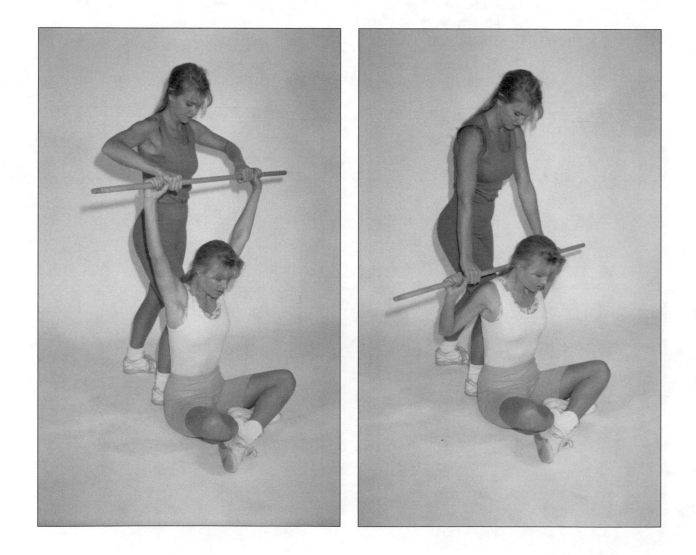

SHOULDER SHRUG

Muscles used: Trapezius.

Starting position: Stand with your arms extended downward, holding a bar or stick. Use an overhand or over and under grip. If a bar is unavailable, your hands can be interlocked.

Description: Keeping your arms straight, shrug your shoulders as high as possible; pause before slowly recovering to the starting position. Repeat the exercise. The resistance should be applied by the body weight of your training partner against the bar.

Point to emphasize:

- If your spotter weighs too much, she should bend her legs to make it easier for you.

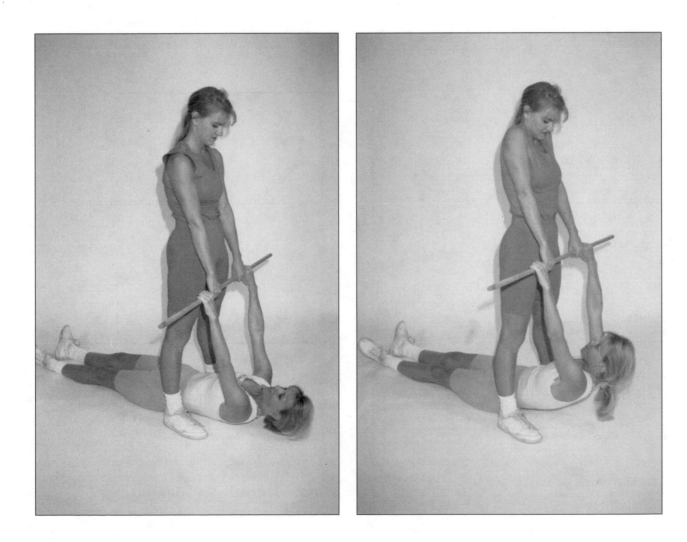

BICEPS CURL

Muscles used: Biceps.

Starting position: Stand with your feet about shoulder-width apart and slightly staggered. Your hands should be at your sides; your palms should be facing forward. Your partner should stand facing you. The bar or wooden dowel should be put in your hands by your partner.

Description: Curl the bar up and toward your chest working against moderate resistance provided by your partner. Once you reach the midrange position of the exercise, you and your partner reverse roles. Your partner forces the bar back to the starting position against moderate resistance provided by you. The first phase of this exercise involves a concentric (positive) movement. The second part involves an eccentric (negative) movement. Repeat the exercise.

Point to emphasize:

- Both movements (the concentric phase and the eccentric phase) should be done slowly, taking 3 to 4 seconds for each direction.

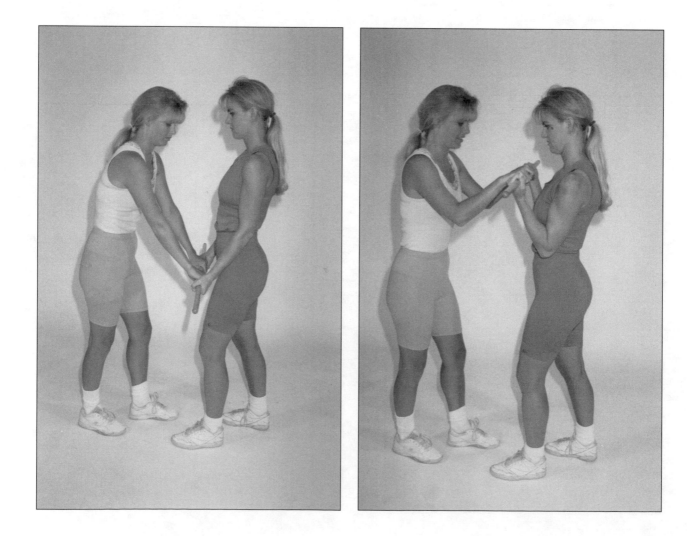

TRICEPS EXTENSION

Muscles used: Triceps.

Starting position: Sit with your legs crossed. Lift your arms overhead, with your elbows pointed skyward, your hands behind your head, and your palms up. Your upper arms should remain as close to your head as possible. The bar or wooden dowel is put in your hands by your partner.

Description: Extend your arms overhead against moderate resistance provided by your partner. Your partner stands behind you and places a knee in your back to give you stability. Once your arms are extended overhead, you and your partner reverse roles. Your partner forces the bar back down to the starting position against resistance provided by you. Note: Overcoming your partner's resistance is a concentric (positive) movement; resisting your partner involves an eccentric (negative) movement.

Point to emphasize:

- Both movements (the concentric phase and the eccentric phase) should be done slowly, taking 3 to 4 seconds for each direction.

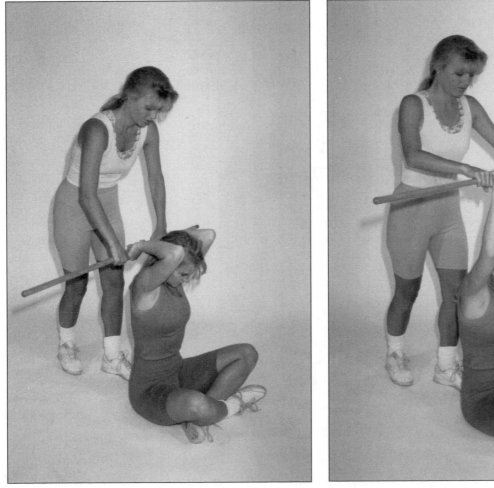
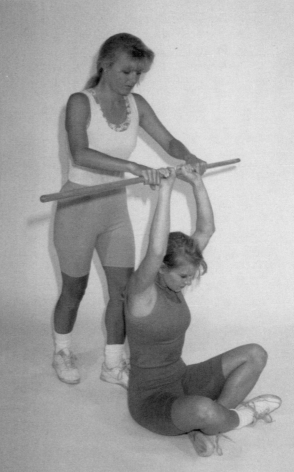

SAMPLE WORKOUTS WITHOUT EQUIPMENT

Workout 1
(Largest to Smallest)

- Leg Press (buddy)
- Leg Curl (buddy)
- Heel Raise (buddy)
- Lat Pulldown/Shoulder Press (stick)
- Back Pulldown/Bench (Chest) Press (stick)
- Front Raise (buddy)
- Shoulder Shrug (stick)
- Triceps Extension (stick)
- Biceps Curl (stick)
- Abdominal Curl (p. 138)

Workout 2
(Push-Pull)

- Leg Press (buddy)
- Leg Curl (buddy)
- Back Pulldown/Bench (Chest) Press (stick)
- Negative-Only Chin-Ups
- Lat Pulldown/Shoulder Press (stick)
- Front Raise (buddy)
- Biceps Curl (stick)
- Triceps Extension (stick)
- Abdominal Curl (p. 138)

Workout 3
(Pre-Exhaustion)

- Hip Adduction (buddy)
- Leg Press (buddy)
- Bent-Arm Fly (buddy)
- Back Pulldown/Bench (Chest) Press (stick)
- Biceps Curl (stick)
- Negative-Only Chin-Ups
- Front Raise (buddy)
- Abdominal Curl (p. 138)

Workout 4
(Upper Body/Lower Body)

- Back Pulldown/Bench (Chest) Press (stick)
- Leg Press (buddy)
- Bent-Over Side Lateral Raise (buddy)
- Hip Abduction (buddy)
- Hip Adduction (buddy)
- Heel Raise (buddy)
- Negative-Only Dips
- Abdominal Curl (p. 138)

PART

III

PUTTING IT ALL TOGETHER

You've set your goals and designed a program to meet them. You've learned the exercises in the four main equipment areas. Now, you're ready to put it all together.

In chapter 8 we offer strength training workouts at the beginner, intermediate, and advanced fitness levels (refer to Assessing Your Strength in chapter 2). We provide these workouts for single set, multiple set, split routine, and circuit training. These exercises can be molded to your special needs and tastes and should serve as a basic starting point from which you can adjust as your strength training needs develop and change.

If you are an athlete training for competitive or recreational sport, turn to chapter 9 for specific workouts for 13 sports. We'll iden-

tify the muscles needed to master the fundamental techniques for each sport, isolate possible problem areas, and show you areas to emphasize. Then you can turn back to chapter 8 and put together a program specific to your sport.

For those of you who simply want to be healthy, look terrific, and feel good about yourself, we've written chapter 10. This chapter presents illustrated beginner, intermediate, and advanced exercises that emphasize those body areas in which women typically experience losses in muscle tone: the stomach, legs, buttocks, and arms.

Let's begin by examining the workouts that provide the foundation for your success.

CHAPTER 8

SAMPLE STRENGTH TRAINING WORKOUTS

This chapter provides sample strength training workouts for the most commonly used programs of strength training—single-set, multiple-set, split routine, and circuit training. Keep in mind that these samples represent only a few of the many possible variations. Let them serve as starting points from which to make adjustments to meet your unique needs and interests. By individualizing your workout, you will enhance its effectiveness and increase your adherence to it.

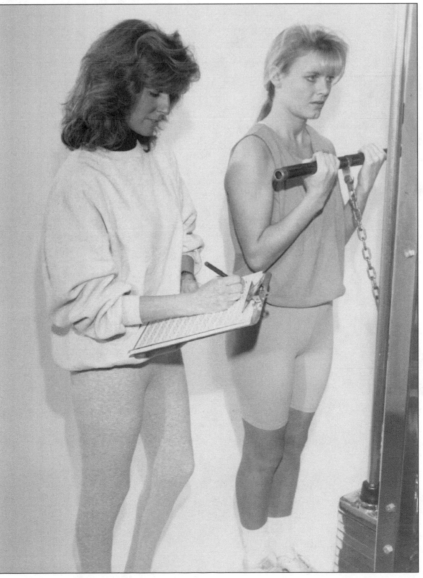

SINGLE-SET PROGRAM

The single-set program, which involves performing each exercise for one set, is an extremely popular method of strength training. Many health and fitness facilities, universities and colleges, and professional sports teams use the single-set method. At West Point, for example, we used it to enhance the muscular fitness capabilities of female and male cadets alike. A single-set program is very effective and viable for people with limited time to devote to strength training.

Sample Single-Set Program Workout (Beginner)

Exercise	Sets	Frequency	Number of Repetitions
Leg Press or Barbell Squat	1	M-W-F	12-15
Leg Curl	1	M-W-F	12-15
Leg Extension	1	M-W-F	12-15
Leg Abduction	1	M-W-F	12-15
Leg Adduction	1	M-W-F	12-15
Heel Raise	1	M-W-F	12-15
Dumbbell Fly	1	M-W-F	12-15
Bench (Chest) Press	1	M-W-F	12-15
Pullover	1	M-W-F	12-15
Lat Pulldown	1	M-W-F	12-15
Side Lateral Raise	1	M-W-F	12-15
Shoulder Press	1	M-W-F	12-15
Biceps Curl	1	M-W-F	12-15
Triceps Extension	1	M-W-F	12-15
Abdominal Curl	1	M-W-F	12-15

Sample Single-Set Program Workout (Intermediate)

Exercise	Sets	Frequency	Number of Repetitions
Leg Press or Barbell Squat	1	M-W-F	8-12
Leg Curl	1	M-W-F	8-12
Leg Extension	1	M-W-F	8-12
Leg Abduction	1	M-W-F	8-12
Leg Adduction	1	M-W-F	8-12
Heel Raise	1	M-W-F	8-12
Dumbbell Fly	1	M-W-F	8-12
Bench (Chest) Press	1	M-W-F	8-12
Pullover	1	M-W-F	8-12
Lat Pulldown	1	M-W-F	8-12
Side Lateral Raise	1	M-W-F	8-12
Shoulder Press	1	M-W-F	8-12
Biceps Curl	1	M-W-F	8-12
Triceps Extension	1	M-W-F	8-12
Abdominal Curl	1	M-W-F	8-12

Sample Single-Set Program Workout (Advanced)

Exercise	Sets	Frequency	Number of Repetitions
Leg Press or Barbell Squat	1	M-W-F	6-10
Leg Curl	1	M-W-F	6-10
Leg Extension	1	M-W-F	6-10
Leg Abduction	1	M-W-F	6-10
Leg Adduction	1	M-W-F	6-10
Heel Raise	1	M-W-F	6-10
Dumbbell Fly	1	M-W-F	6-10
Bench (Chest) Press	1	M-W-F	6-10
Pullover	1	M-W-F	6-10
Lat Pulldown	1	M-W-F	6-10
Side Lateral Raise	1	M-W-F	6-10
Shoulder Press	1	M-W-F	6-10
Biceps Curl	1	M-W-F	6-10
Triceps Extension	1	M-W-F	6-10
Abdominal Curl	1	M-W-F	6-10

MULTIPLE-SET PROGRAM

In a multiple-set program you perform each exercise for several sets. We recommend two or three sets depending on your level of training experience. The more advanced exerciser, for example, should do three sets of each exercise with relatively heavy loads. The multiple-set program has been popular since the 1940s, and many of today's widely used programs are variations. This approach to strength training requires more time than the single-set program.

Sample Multiple-Set Program Workout (Beginner)

Exercise	Sets	Frequency	Number of Repetitions
Leg Press or Barbell Squat	2	M-W-F	12-15
Leg Curl	2	M-W-F	12-15
Leg Extension	2	M-W-F	12-15
Leg Abduction	2	M-W-F	12-15
Leg Adduction	2	M-W-F	12-15
Heel Raise	2	M-W-F	12-15
Dumbbell Fly	2	M-W-F	12-15
Bench (Chest) Press	2	M-W-F	12-15
Pullover	2	M-W-F	12-15
Lat Pulldown	2	M-W-F	12-15
Side Lateral Raise	2	M-W-F	12-15
Shoulder Press	2	M-W-F	12-15
Biceps Curl	2	M-W-F	12-15
Triceps Extension	2	M-W-F	12-15
Abdominal Curl	2	M-W-F	12-15

Sample Multiple-Set Program Workout (Intermediate)

Exercise	Sets	Frequency	Number of Repetitions
Leg Press or Barbell Squat	3	M-W-F	8-12
Leg Curl	3	M-W-F	8-12
Leg Extension	3	M-W-F	8-12
Leg Abduction	3	M-W-F	8-12
Leg Adduction	3	M-W-F	8-12
Heel Raise	3	M-W-F	8-12
Dumbbell Fly	3	M-W-F	8-12
Bench (Chest) Press	3	M-W-F	8-12
Pullover	3	M-W-F	8-12
Lat Pulldown	3	M-W-F	8-12
Side Lateral Raise	3	M-W-F	8-12
Shoulder Press	3	M-W-F	8-12
Biceps Curl	3	M-W-F	8-12
Triceps Extension	3	M-W-F	8-12
Abdominal Curl	3	M-W-F	8-12

Sample Multiple-Set Program Workout (Advanced)

Exercise	Sets	Frequency	Number of Repetitions
Leg Press or Barbell Squat	3	M-W-F	5-8
Leg Curl	3	M-W-F	5-8
Leg Extension	3	M-W-F	5-8
Leg Abduction	3	M-W-F	5-8
Leg Adduction	3	M-W-F	5-8
Heel Raise	3	M-W-F	5-8
Dumbbell Fly	3	M-W-F	5-8
Bench (Chest) Press	3	M-W-F	5-8
Lat Pullover	3	M-W-F	5-8
Lat Pulldown	3	M-W-F	5-8
Side Lateral Raise	3	M-W-F	5-8
Shoulder Press	3	M-W-F	5-8
Biceps Curl	3	M-W-F	5-8
Triceps Extension	3	M-W-F	5-8
Abdominal Curl	3	M-W-F	5-8

SPLIT ROUTINE PROGRAM

A split routine program involves training different body parts on alternate days. A typical split routine program might be training your chest, back, and shoulders Monday, Wednesday, and Friday, and your legs, arms, and abdominal region Tuesday, Thursday, and Saturday. A split routine program is popular among bodybuilders, since they believe it's necessary to do many exercises for a body part to get improvements in muscular size. It's important to remember that, even though you work out 6 days a week, a split routine program is designed to give enough rebuilding time for the muscle groups exercised, because the same body parts aren't trained on successive days.

Sample Split Routine Program Workout (Beginner)

Exercise	Sets	Frequency	Number of Repetitions
Leg Press or Barbell Squat	1	T-Th-S	8-12
Leg Curl	1	T-Th-S	8-12
Leg Extension	1	T-Th-S	8-12
Leg Abduction	1	T-Th-S	8-12
Leg Adduction	1	T-Th-S	8-12
Heel Raise	1	T-Th-S	8-12
Biceps Curl	1	T-Th-S	8-12
Triceps Extension	1	T-Th-S	8-12
Abdominal Curl	1	T-Th-S	8-12
Dumbbell Fly	1	M-W-F	8-12
Bench (Chest) Press	1	M-W-F	8-12
Pullover	1	M-W-F	8-12
Lat Pulldown	1	M-W-F	8-12
Side Lateral Raise	1	M-W-F	8-12
Shoulder Press	1	M-W-F	8-12

Sample Split Routine Program Workout (Intermediate)

Exercise	Sets	Frequency	Number of Repetitions
Leg Press or Barbell Squat	2	T-Th-S	8-12
Leg Curl	2	T-Th-S	8-12
Leg Extension	2	T-Th-S	8-12
Leg Abduction	2	T-Th-S	8-12
Leg Adduction	2	T-Th-S	8-12
Heel Raise	2	T-Th-S	8-12
Biceps Curl	2	T-Th-S	8-12
Triceps Extension	2	T-Th-S	8-12
Abdominal Curl	2	T-Th-S	8-12
Dumbbell Fly	2	M-W-F	8-12
Chest Press	2	M-W-F	8-12
Pullover	2	M-W-F	8-12
Lat Pulldown	2	M-W-F	8-12
Side Lateral Raise	2	M-W-F	8-12
Shoulder Press	2	M-W-F	8-12

Sample Split Routine Program Workout (Advanced)

Exercise	Sets	Frequency	Number of Repetitions
Leg Press or Barbell Squat	3	T-Th-S	8-12
Leg Curl	3	T-Th-S	8-12
Leg Extension	3	T-Th-S	8-12
Leg Abduction	3	T-Th-S	8-12
Leg Adduction	3	T-Th-S	8-12
Heel Raise	3	T-Th-S	8-12
Biceps Curl	3	T-Th-S	8-12
Triceps Extension	3	T-Th-S	8-12
Abdominal Curl	3	T-Th-S	8-12
Dumbbell Fly	3	M-W-F	8-12
Bench (Chest) Press	3	M-W-F	8-12
Pullover	3	M-W-F	8-12
Lat Pulldown	3	M-W-F	8-12
Side Lateral Raise	3	M-W-F	8-12
Shoulder Press	3	M-W-F	8-12

CIRCUIT TRAINING PROGRAM

The goal of circuit training is to simultaneously improve aerobic fitness and muscular strength and endurance. While circuit training has a positive effect on muscular fitness, it gives only a modest improvement in aerobic fitness.

Circuit training programs usually have 6 to 15 strength training stations per circuit (see Figure 8.1). The circuit is repeated 2 or 3 times so the total exercise time is about 20 to 30 minutes. Little or no rest should be taken between exercise stations.

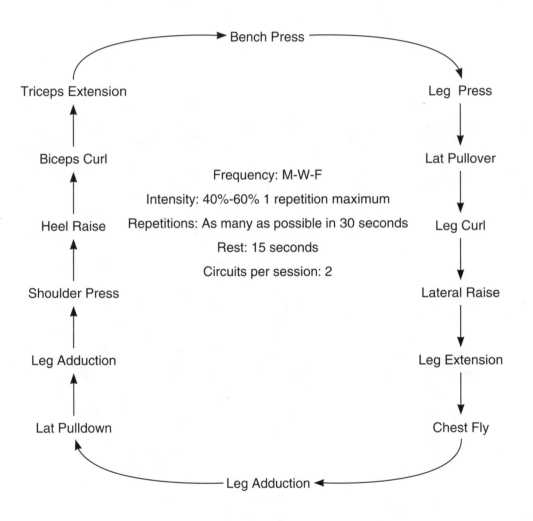

Frequency: M-W-F

Intensity: 40%-60% 1 repetition maximum

Repetitions: As many as possible in 30 seconds

Rest: 15 seconds

Circuits per session: 2

Figure 8.1a   Sample circuit training program workout (beginner).

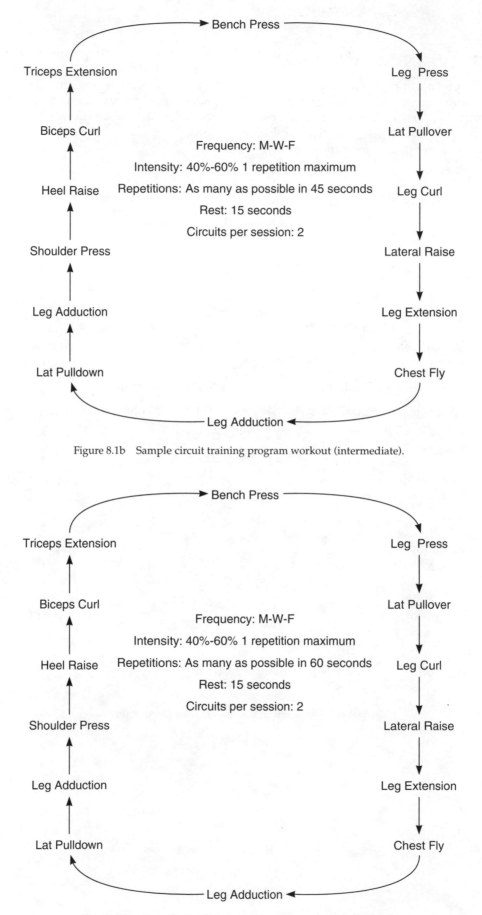

Figure 8.1b   Sample circuit training program workout (intermediate).

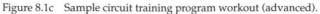

Figure 8.1c   Sample circuit training program workout (advanced).

CHAPTER 9
STRENGTH TRAINING FOR SPORTS

To a certain extent, great athletes are born, not made. In that regard, the best thing a want-to-be superstar could do would be to choose her parents wisely. Despite the extravagant claims made for this particular workout program or that particular wonder drug, all athletes are "blessed" or "cursed" with characteristics that no barbell, exercise regimen, or dietary supplement can change.

As we discussed in chapter 1, a higher level of muscular fitness will provide you with at least two fundamental benefits: reduced injury potential and enhanced performance potential. While these effects can help women of all ages and interests, they are very important to those who play sports. Given the dynamic, volatile nature of ath-

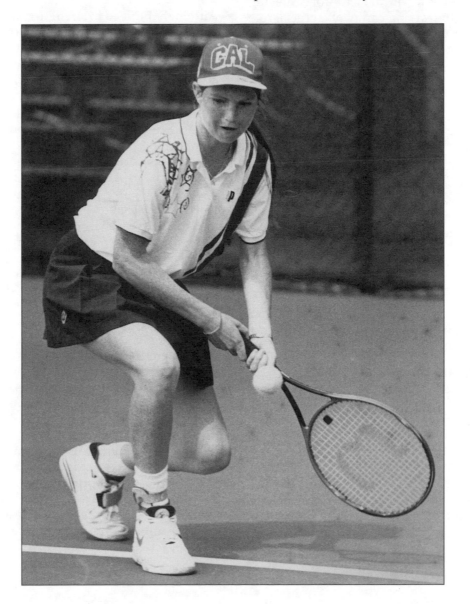

letics, you could be exposed to a high risk of injury during a contest. Uncontrolled motion, external forces, sudden stops, immovable objects, and above-average velocity are a few factors that can result in an athlete being injured. If you increase the fitness level of a muscle and its connective tissues (tendons and ligaments), you will be less endangered by these risks. As an athlete, you should view strength training as a sound and inexpensive form of health insurance.

You should also consider how resistance training can enhance your performance. A higher level of muscular fitness will not only increase your fatigue threshold, but also enable the muscle to recover more quickly and efficiently. As the great former basketball coach of UCLA, John Wooden, once said: "In any close contest, in any sport, conditioning will be the key to victory." Having your muscles ready and able to do what you want at any moment can be a critical factor for achieving success. Strength training can play a crucial role in determining whether your muscles "can do" or have to "make do."

FUNCTION AT THE JUNCTION

In addition to genetic factors and a well-designed and implemented conditioning program, your ability to perform selected motor functions influences how well you do athletically. Collectively, these functions are defined as motor ability. Individually, each plays a role in athletic performance (definitions of the basic motor functions follow). For many athletes, a high level of ability in these motor functions can make a difference between success and failure. To a limited extent, you can affect your ability in the motor functions through conditioning (particularly strength training because each function involves movement) and practice (resulting in a higher level of neuromuscular efficiency).

Definitions of the Basic Motor Functions

Agility—is your ability to change directions rapidly and effectively while moving at a high rate of speed.

Balance—is your ability to maintain a specific body position while either stationary or moving.

Coordination—is the smooth, desired flow of movement in the execution of a motor task. Forceful and explosive movements are blended with accurate and less forceful movements to achieve purposeful movement.

Kinesthetic sense—is your ability to be aware of the positions of various parts of your body. It is particularly important in athletics.

Movement time—is the time required to move part of your body from one point to another.

Reaction time—is the time required for you to initiate a response to a stimulus.

Response time—is movement time plus reaction time.

Speed—is the time required to move your body from one place to another.

ATHLETIC PROGRAM CONSIDERATIONS

Although the need to strength train may be more obvious for athletes than nonathletes, the approach and techniques for the two groups are essentially the same. How you develop a muscle doesn't change because you're an athlete. The fundamentals, techniques, and principles outlined in chapter 2 are as important to the nonathlete as to the sportswoman.

Two issues that athletes must consider, which may or may not apply to nonathletes, are the need for seasonal program adjustments and the need to develop the muscles that are involved in your sport. Most strength training programs for athletes include seasonal adjustments in their design. For example, many athletes strength train twice a week during the season and three times a week during the off-season. Other athletes cut back on the number of exercises performed during an in-season workout. In the interest of conserving time, some split their workouts during the season (upper body exercises one day and lower body exercises the next, instead of whole body workouts on nonconsecutive days). As a rule, the intensity of the workouts remains the same. Only the net amount of exercise is diminished. Whatever your preference, you shouldn't strength train for 36 hours before competing.

Ensure that your resistance training program includes exercises to develop the musculature involved in your sport. The first step is to identify what muscles are involved in what sport. Table 9.1 provides a list of muscle groups used in popular athletic activities. Figure 9.1 shows the anterior and posterior muscles of the body.

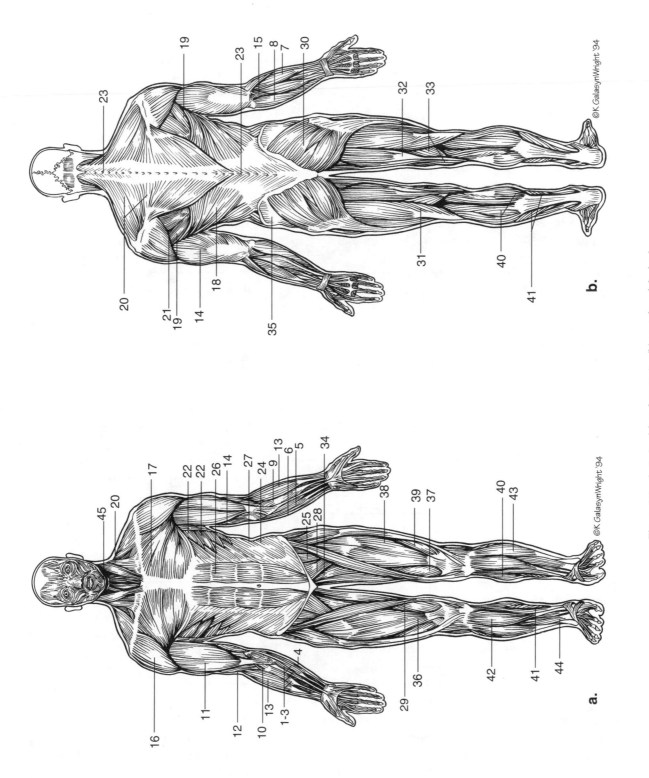

Figure 9.1   Anterior (a) and posterior (b) muscles of the body.

Table 9.1   Muscle Involvement in Sports

Muscle	Action Numbers in ( ) indicate muscles that assist in action	Sport In which greatest resistance is encountered
1. Flexor digitorum profundus 2. Flexor digitorum sublimis	Closes fingers	Any sport in which one grasps an opponent, partner, or equipment, such as hand-to-hand balancing, tennis, horizontal bar, batting
3. Flexor pollicis longus	Flexes thumb	
4. Palmaris longus 5. Flexor carpi radialis 6. Flexor carpi ulnaris	Flexes wrist palmward and to both sides (1,2,3,7,8)	Tennis, throwing a softball, handball, two-handed pass in basketball, batting, golf swing
7. Extensor carpi radialis longus and brevis 8. Extensor carpi ulnaris	Extends wrist	Backhand stroke in tennis and badminton, Olympic weight lifting, bait and fly casting
9. Pronator teres	Pronates forearm	Tennis forehand, shot put, throwing a punch, throwing a baseball, passing a football
10. Supinator	Supinates forearm (11)	Throwing a curve ball, batting, fencing thrust
11. Biceps brachii 12. Brachialis	Flexes elbow (9)	Ring work, rope climb, archery, back stroke in swimming
13. Brachioradialis	Flexes elbow strongly when forearm is pronated or partially pronated	Rowing, cleaning a barbell, rope climbing
14. Triceps brachii 15. Anconeus	Extends elbow	Breaststroke, shot put, parallel bar work, vaulting, hand shivers in football, hand balancing, batting, pole vaulting, fencing thrust, passing a basketball
16. Deltoid (For simplicity this muscle is divided into anterior and posterior fibers only.)	Anterior fibers—adducts, elevates, inwardly rotates humerus Posterior fibers—abducts, depresses, outwardly rotates humerus	Hand balancing, canoeing, shot put, pole vaulting, tennis, archery, batting, fencing thrust, breaststroke, back- and crawl strokes, golf swing, handball

Muscle	Action	Sport
17. Pectoralis major	Elevates humerus forward (16) Adducts humerus (16,19) Depresses humerus (16,18,19); inwardly rotates humerus (18,19)	Crawl and backstrokes, tennis, throwing a softball, shot put, discus throw, straight arm lever position in gymnastics
18. Latissimus dorsi 19. Teres major	Draws humerus down and backward (16); inwardly rotates humerus (16,17)	Rope climb; canoe racing; ring work; rowing; batting; crawl, back-, breast-, and butterfly strokes; golf swing
20. Trapezius	A. Tilts head back (23) B. Elevates shoulder point C. Adducts scapula	A. Gymnastic bridge B. Cleaning a barbell, breast stroke C. Archery, batting, breast stroke
21. Rhomboids, major and minor	Adducts scapula (20)	Tennis backhand, batting, back- and breaststrokes
22. Serratus anterior	Abducts scapula	Shot put, discus throw, tennis, archery, tackling, crawl
23. Erector spinae (also includes a number of smaller groups)	Extends spine (20) Laterally flexes spine (20,26,27) Rotates spine	Discus throw, batting, golf swing, racing start in swimming, diving, tumbling, rowing
24. External oblique 25. Internal oblique 26. Rectus abdominis 27. Transversalis	Flexes spine Laterally flexes spine (23) Rotates spine (23) Compresses abdomen	This group of muscles is important in all sports. Posture, general fitness, and appearance cannot be overstated.
28. Iliopsoas	Flexes trunk (27) Flexes thigh (36)	Running, hurdling, pole vaulting, kicking a soccer ball, flutter kick, pike and tuck positions in tumbling and diving
29. Sartorius	Flexes femur (39) Flexes knee Rotates femur outward	Tumbling and diving
30. Gluteus maximus	Extends femur (31,32,33) Rotates femur outward (31)	Skiing, shot put, running, quick starts in track, all jumping and skipping, skating, swimming start, changing direction while running

(continued)

Table 9.1   (*continued*)

Muscle	Action	Sport
31. Biceps femoris	Extends femur (30) Flexes knee (40) Rotates femur outward (30)	Skiing, skating, quick starts in track and swimming, hurdling, line play, all jumping
32. Semitendinosus 33. Semimembranosus	Flexes knee (40) Extends femur (30) Rotates femur inward	
34. Adductor magnus	Adducts femur and rotates outward during adduction	Skiing, skating, frog kick, bareback horseback riding
35. Gluteus medius	Abducts femur (essential for spring)	Hurdling, fencing, frog kick, shot put, running, skating
36. Rectus femoris	Flexes femur (28) Extends knee	
37. Vastus internus 38. Vastus intermedius 39. Vastus externus	Extends knee	Skiing, skating, quick starts, all jumping, kick in soccer, flutter kick, frog kick, water skiing, diving, trampoline and tumbling, bicycling, catching in softball
40. Gastrocnemius	Extends foot when knee is almost straight (44)	Quick starts in track, swimming, basketball, football, skating, all jumping, skiing
41. Soleus	Extends foot when knee is bent	
42. Tibialis anterior	Flexes and inverts foot	Changing direction while running, skating, skiing
43. Peroneus longus	Extends foot (40,41,44) Inverts foot	Skating turns, changing direction while running
44. Flexor hallucis longs	Flexes big toe Extends ankle	Running, all jumping, racing starts
45. Sternomastoid	Tucks chin Rotates head Raises sternum in deep breathing	Crawl stroke, tucking chin in diving, football, boxing, distance running (breathing)

• Reprinted by permission of Cramer Products, Inc.

STRENGTH TRAINING PROGRAMS

In the following pages, we provide an overview of the developmental strength needs for 13 selected sports. Identify what strength training exercises will develop each muscle (see Table 2.3), and include the appropriate exercises in your program.

STRENGTH TRAINING FOR BASKETBALL

FUNDAMENTAL TECHNIQUES:

Basic Skills	Muscles Involved
1. Jumping	Buttocks, quadriceps, hamstrings
2. Throwing	Latissimus dorsi, deltoids, pectorals, triceps
3. Rebounding	Buttocks, quadriceps, hamstrings, biceps, forearm flexors
4. Dribbling	Hand-wrist flexors
5. Shooting	Deltoids, triceps, pectorals, forearm flexors and extensors, hand flexors and extensors

POTENTIAL PROBLEM AREAS:

- Knees, ankles
- Shoulders
- Aerobic capacity (stamina)
- Muscle fatigue

AREAS TO EMPHASIZE:

- Develop the forearm flexors and the biceps to increase grip strength for holding on to the ball and pulling it away from an opponent.
- Develop the muscles used for shooting so shooting ability won't be easily affected by muscular fatigue.
- Strengthen the knee to decrease its susceptibility to injury.

STRENGTH TRAINING FOR FIELD HOCKEY

FUNDAMENTAL TECHNIQUES:

Basic Skills	Muscles Involved
1. Running	Quadriceps, hamstrings, buttocks
2. Stickwork—passing and receiving	Latissimus dorsi, deltoids, triceps, pectorals, biceps
3. Shooting	Latissimus dorsi, pectorals, deltoids, triceps

POTENTIAL PROBLEM AREAS:

- Stamina
- Grip strength
- Muscular fatigue
- Knee injuries

AREAS TO EMPHASIZE:

- Develop the forearm and hand flexors to strengthen your grip.
- Develop the arm and shoulder muscles used for shooting and stick handling to decrease the severity of muscular fatigue.
- Develop the leg muscles so that violent collisions won't result in knee injuries.

STRENGTH TRAINING FOR GOLF

FUNDAMENTAL TECHNIQUES:

Basic Skills	Muscles Involved
1. Driving power	Buttocks, quadriceps, hamstrings, lower back muscles
2. Hip/body turn	Lower back muscles, hip flexors, obliques
3. Impact velocity	Latissimus dorsi, triceps
4. Club extension	Deltoids, triceps
5. Clubhead control	Triceps, biceps, forearm and hand flexors
6. Walking endurance	Buttocks, quadriceps

POTENTIAL PROBLEM AREAS:

- Muscular fatigue
- Hand injuries (blisters, etc.)
- Walking stamina
- Joint aches and discomfort

AREAS TO EMPHASIZE:

- Develop the forearm and hand flexors to protect your hands and wrists from injuries.
- Develop the muscles used in the golf swing to delay or prevent muscular fatigue.
- Include flexibility exercises regularly.
- Warm up properly.

STRENGTH TRAINING FOR GYMNASTICS

FUNDAMENTAL TECHNIQUES:

Basic Skills	Muscles Involved
1. Vaulting	Buttocks, quadriceps, lower back
2. Pressing movement (e.g., parallel bars)	Deltoids, triceps, pectorals
3. Pulling movement	Latissimus dorsi, biceps
4. Straight arm lever (e.g., hand balance)	Pectorals, deltoids
5. Trampoline and tumbling	Iliopsoas, sartorius
6. Floor exercise	Buttocks, lower back, quadriceps, deltoids, triceps, pectorals

POTENTIAL PROBLEM AREAS:

- Muscular fatigue
- Muscular soreness
- Flexibility
- Shoulder and ankle injuries

AREAS TO EMPHASIZE:

- Develop the muscles used for gymnastic skills to prevent muscular fatigue.

- Develop joint (ankle, knee, shoulder) stability to minimize injuries.
- Include flexibility exercises regularly.
- Warm up thoroughly.

STRENGTH TRAINING FOR MARTIAL ARTS

FUNDAMENTAL TECHNIQUES:

Basic Skills	Muscles Involved
1. Methods of holding	Flexor pollicis longus, palmaris longus
2. Methods of unbalancing	Flexor digitorum profundus
3. Hand throws	Biceps, rectus abdominis
4. Hip throws	Quadriceps, scalenus
5. Leg throws	Gastrocnemius, hamstrings
6. Back and side throws	Deltoids
7. Grappling techniques	Pectorals
8. Strangling holds	Latissimus dorsi, biceps, deltoids
9. Armlock techniques	Biceps, triceps, trapezius

POTENTIAL PROBLEM AREAS:

- Ankles
- Fingers
- Neck
- Weak shoulders
- Wrists
- Arms (about the elbow)

AREAS TO EMPHASIZE:

- Develop overall body musculature to delay muscular fatigue.
- Maintain an aerobic program for stamina.
- Develop your upper torso muscles.
- Emphasize flexibility and joint stability exercises to reduce injuries.

STRENGTH TRAINING FOR RACQUETBALL AND SQUASH

FUNDAMENTAL TECHNIQUES:

Basic Skills	Muscles Involved
1. Running, cutting movements	Buttocks, lower back, quadriceps, hamstrings
2. Hitting the ball	Pectorals, triceps, biceps, latissimus dorsi
3. Wrist control	Hand and forearm flexors

POTENTIAL PROBLEM AREAS:

- Stamina
- Muscular fatigue
- Grip strength
- Elbow and shoulder injuries

AREAS TO EMPHASIZE:

- Implement an aerobic program for stamina.
- Develop the muscles used for racquetball to delay muscular fatigue.
- Emphasize joint stability and flexibility exercises to reduce the possibility of injuries.
- Develop grip strength to improve racquet control.
- Warm up properly.

STRENGTH TRAINING FOR RUNNING

FUNDAMENTAL TECHNIQUES:

Basic Skills	Muscles Involved
1. Running, striding	Quadriceps, buttocks, calves, lower back, hamstrings, hip flexors
2. Stabilizing the torso	Latissimus dorsi, abdominals, obliques
3. Stabilizing the shoulder girdle	Deltoids, trapezius

POTENTIAL PROBLEM AREAS:

- Stamina
- Muscular fatigue
- Foot injuries
- Knees, hips, ankles

AREAS TO EMPHASIZE:

- Maintain an aerobic program for stamina.
- Develop the muscles used for running to delay muscular fatigue.
- Emphasize joint stability and flexibility exercises.
- Warm up properly.

STRENGTH TRAINING FOR SKIING

FUNDAMENTAL TECHNIQUES:

Basic Skills	Muscles Involved
1. Maintaining weight over skis	Quadriceps, buttocks, hamstrings
2. Absorbing shock of landings	Quadriceps, buttocks, hamstrings
3. Driving off poles	Deltoids, triceps, latissimus dorsi
4. Maintaining balance	Quadriceps, hamstrings, lower back

POTENTIAL PROBLEM AREAS:

- Muscular endurance
- Stamina
- Knee injuries
- Ankle injuries

AREAS TO EMPHASIZE:

- Develop musculature involved in the basic skills of skiing.
- Develop stamina using a comprehensive running/interval training.
- Develop joint stability through strength conditioning of muscles surrounding susceptible joints.
- Emphasize flexibility exercises.

STRENGTH TRAINING FOR SOCCER

FUNDAMENTAL TECHNIQUES:

Basic Skills	Muscles Involved
1. Kicking	Buttocks, quadriceps, lower back, gastrocnemius
2. Heading the ball	Trapezius, neck extensors and flexors
3. Running	Buttocks, hamstrings, quadriceps, lower back
4. In-bounding the ball	Latissimus dorsi, deltoid, triceps
5. Catching and gripping the ball (goalie only)	Forearm flexors, deltoid, triceps

POTENTIAL PROBLEM AREAS:

- Stamina
- Muscular fatigue
- Lower leg injuries
- Neck injuries

AREAS TO EMPHASIZE:

- Develop stamina (wind) with an extensive aerobic conditioning program.
- Develop the muscles used in soccer to delay muscular fatigue.
- Emphasize the neck and lower legs in your muscle development program to minimize injuries.
- Emphasize flexibility and joint stability exercises.
- Warm up properly.

STRENGTH TRAINING FOR SOFTBALL

FUNDAMENTAL TECHNIQUES:

Basic Skills	Muscles Involved
1. Hitting	Buttocks, lead arm triceps, forearm flexors, pectorals, latissimus dorsi, deltoids, triceps
2. Running	Quadriceps, buttocks, hamstrings
3. Throwing	Buttocks, quadriceps, hamstrings, obliques, abdominals, lower pectorals, deltoids, rhomboids, latissimus dorsi, triceps, forearm flexors, biceps
4. Catching	Forearm flexors, deltoids, latissimus dorsi

POTENTIAL PROBLEM AREAS:

- Knees, ankles
- Shoulders
- Elbows
- Muscle fatigue

AREAS TO EMPHASIZE:

- Develop your forearm flexors for grip control.
- Develop your upper back (latissimus dorsi), which is the primary muscle in the upper body used for throwing.
- Develop your upper arm (biceps and triceps) to minimize the possibility of hyperextending or jamming the elbow joint while throwing.

STRENGTH TRAINING FOR SWIMMING

FUNDAMENTAL TECHNIQUES:

Basic Skills	Muscles Involved
1. Starting	Buttocks, lower back, quadriceps
2. Turning	Buttocks, lower back, hamstrings, quadriceps
3. Kicking	Buttocks, lower back, quadriceps
4. All strokes	Latissimus dorsi, pectorals, deltoids, triceps, biceps, trapezius, abdominals

POTENTIAL PROBLEM AREAS:

- Muscular fatigue
- Stamina

- Flexibility
- Abdominals

AREAS TO EMPHASIZE:

- Develop the muscles used for each stroke to delay muscular fatigue.
- Include prolonged exercise in the water to develop aerobic endurance.
- Emphasize flexibility exercises to maximize stroke efficiency and reduce joint-related injuries.
- Develop your abdominals as much as possible.

STRENGTH TRAINING FOR TENNIS

FUNDAMENTAL TECHNIQUES:

Basic Skills	Muscles Involved
1. Running	Buttocks, quadriceps, hamstrings
2. Serving	Deltoids, triceps, biceps, latissimus dorsi, trapezius, obliques
3. Forehand	Latissimus dorsi, biceps, triceps, forearm flexors, obliques
4. Backhand	Triceps, biceps, deltoids, latissimus dorsi, forearm flexors, obliques
5. Racquet control	Forearm flexors, triceps, biceps

POTENTIAL PROBLEM AREAS:

- Muscular fatigue
- Stamina
- Tennis elbow
- Lower back and shoulder injuries

AREAS TO EMPHASIZE:

- Develop stamina using a comprehensive running/interval program.

- Develop the musculature involved in the basic tennis skills.
- Increase joint stability by developing the muscles that facilitate joint movement.

STRENGTH TRAINING FOR VOLLEYBALL

FUNDAMENTAL TECHNIQUES:

Basic Skills	Muscles Involved
1. Jumping	Buttocks, quadriceps, hamstrings
2. Serving	Deltoids, trapezius, latissimus dorsi
3. Setting	Pectorals, deltoids, triceps, biceps
4. Spiking	Deltoids, triceps, forearm flexors, latissimus dorsi
5. Digging	Biceps, latissimus dorsi, trapezius, pectorals
6. Blocking	Deltoids, latissimus dorsi, trapezius
7. Sprinting	Buttocks, quadriceps, hamstrings, adductors, abductors

POTENTIAL PROBLEM AREAS:

- Muscular endurance
- Stamina
- Shoulder injuries
- Leg muscle strains

AREAS TO EMPHASIZE:

- Use a comprehensive running/interval program to develop stamina.
- Develop muscles that are critical to the performance of basic volleyball skills.
- Emphasize flexibility conditioning.
- Develop musculature of the shoulder girdle and legs.
- Develop knee joint stability.

CHAPTER 10

FIRMING UP YOUR BODY: THE FIT LOOK

We all want to be healthy, look terrific, and feel good about ourselves, so most of us are conscious about our appearance. We want our appearance to be compatible with how we think we should look. Loosely translated, we all want to look "fit."

What is the fit look? A fit body has several characteristics. It's usually firm and relatively hard. It often belongs to OTHER people. A fit body allows you to wear the desired clothes without worrying about how well they can hide bulges. If your body is fit, you may get a kind word from your family physician during your annual physical. Above all, a fit body will contribute to your physical and mental well-being. Beauty, as the adage goes, is in the eye of the beholder. If you feel good about yourself, that's super. That's what this chapter is about—feeling good and looking terrific.

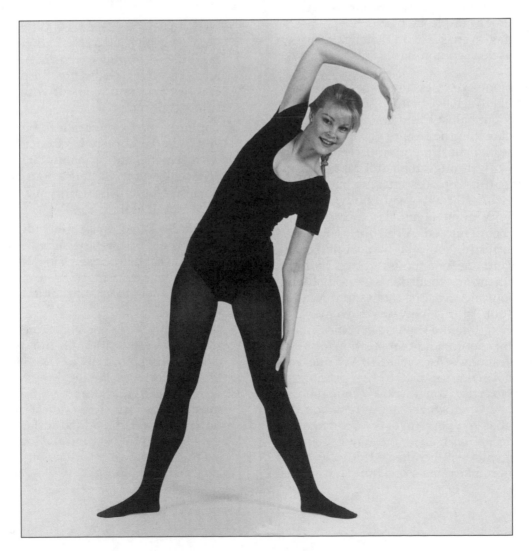

THE EXERCISES

Although you may be in good physical condition, you may not have that fit look. Some areas of your body may be flabby and lacking firmness and muscle tone. The exercises in this chapter are designed to firm, shape, and contour muscles. Although these exercises won't result in spot reducing or massive losses in body weight, muscle toning exercises will improve your girth measurements. This will enhance the fit of your clothing and move you closer to that fit look. These exercises won't add bulk to your muscles. They will, however, have a positive effect on your appearance and your level of fitness. Natural feminine curves are most attractive when they are supported by firm, toned underlying muscles.

The exercises in this chapter emphasize body areas where women typically experience loss in muscle tone: stomach or abdominal muscles, legs, buttocks, and arms. Although muscle toning exercises can firm and reshape your body for that fit look, they will not change your individual body type. For example, no matter how hard she works, toning exercises won't change a stocky, heavily muscled woman into a thin, or slender one.

Muscle toning exercises should be done slowly and smoothly to achieve better results. Fast, jerky movements are ballistic and counterproductive to safely achieving the results you want. When you exercise ballistically, your muscles aren't required to work through their full range of motion. Momentum replaces effective muscle actions. You will be throwing your body, not exercising it. Jerky movements also increase your chances of being injured. A rule for doing these exercises correctly would be two counts (count "one thousand one, one thousand two") for upward movement, and four counts ("one thousand one, one thousand two, one thousand three, one thousand four") for downward movement. In addition, each time the exercise specifies a held position, you should hold that position for 2 to 3 seconds unless otherwise specified. As a rule, you should perform one set of 10 to 12 repetitions of a particular exercise. You can do a second set, also of 10 to 12 reps. However many reps you do, make sure that you perform every one properly. If you try to do too many, you may get sloppy and your results will be affected. Ideally, these exercises should be done 4 or 5 times a week. At the minimum, you should work out 3 times a week if you want noticeable results.

For each of the four areas of your body, exercises are presented for three levels of difficulty: beginner, intermediate, and advanced. The beginner's exercises are for the person who is just starting an exercise program; the intermediate ones are for someone who has been doing some form of regular exercise or physical activity; and the advanced exercises are for the person who exercises vigorously almost every day. With regular exercise, you should notice improvements within 4 to 6 weeks. Improvements will occur, however, only if you do the exercises properly and regularly. Because of each person's unique characteristics, the same muscle toning exercises may affect body measurements differently from person to person. Research and experience have shown that muscle tone improvement depends on your desire and the effort you put into your program. If your desire and training effort are both high, your fit look may be only weeks away.

Follow these exercise guidelines:

- As with any new exercise program, check with your physician about your plans to do these muscle toning exercises. Also, if an injury occurs or you become ill during your exercise program, consult your physician before continuing.

- For any exercise program to be successful, you must combine your exercise program with sensible eating habits. It's foolish to believe that you can abuse your body nutritionally and still firm up your muscles or have that fit look.

- What time you exercise is an individual matter. It would be wise to wait at least an hour after you eat before exercising. Research has shown that exercising at the same time each day helps you to establish it as a consistent habit.

- What you wear when you exercise is a personal decision. Although trendy workout clothes may be fun, all you need is loose-fitting, comfortable clothing. Exercise in a large, well-ventilated area, and try to exercise to music or a favorite television show. Exercise on a rug, towel, or padded surface to protect your body from irritation and bruises. These exercises shouldn't be done on a bed or an extremely soft surface.

- If possible, exercise with a buddy so that you can motivate and support each other. Also, it's much harder to opt out of the commitment to exercise if it involves another person.

- If you are unaccustomed to physical activity and muscle toning exercise in particular, start your program gradually with the beginner exercises. Don't overwork muscle groups—you should only experience moderate muscle fatigue. Mild muscle soreness, however, isn't unusual during the first few weeks of exercising. If you do get sore, continue exercising, but at a slower rate and for less time. If the soreness lasts more than a few days, either the intensity of your program is too high or you may have a medical problem that requires attention. A warm bath or shower may also be relaxing and helpful to ease soreness.

- Try to do muscle toning exercises 4 or 5 times a week. If you exercise regularly, you should see improvements in 4 to 6 weeks. The more you exercise, the quicker your improvement will be. Be patient, however. You didn't get out of shape and lose tone overnight, and you won't get that fit look overnight.

- Breathe normally and freely while exercising. Never hold your breath.

- Be careful not to arch (hyperextend) your back while doing exercises that involve your lower back. Always try to keep your lower back extended, and when appropriate, in contact with the floor. Most of the toning exercises described in this chapter are done from a seated or floor position rather than standing. This is because seated or prone exercises place less strain on your lower back. Because millions of people suffer from back problems, it's important to protect your back as much as possible while exercising.

- Finally, warm-up activities that increase circulation and raise muscle temperature should be done at the beginning of every exercise program. Warm-ups prepare you for more strenuous activity and help to prevent injuries. Do at least 5 minutes of stretching and slow-moving activities. Do your warm-ups slowly and smoothly; don't jerk or bounce. Try some slow arm circles, leg swings, running in place, or old-fashioned jumping jacks as warm-up activities.

STOMACH (ABDOMINALS)

Beginning Level

1. **Single-Leg Lift:** Lie on your back with your arms out at your shoulders. Bring your right knee to your chest, extend your leg up toward the ceiling (toes pointed), return it to your chest, and then to the floor. Repeat with your left leg, right, left, in succession.

2. **Curl:** Lie on your back with your knees bent and your hands on your shoulders. Slowly curl your head forward, tucking your chin to your chest. Continue to curl up until your head and shoulders are off the floor about 12 to 15 in. Pause, then slowly curl down to the floor. Relax and repeat. Be sure to breathe freely throughout the exercise. If you have difficulty doing the exercise with your hands resting on your shoulders, extend your hands forward and reach toward your knees while you are curling up.

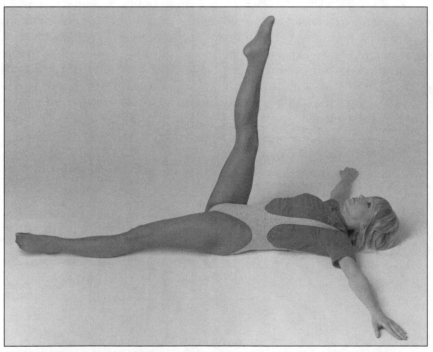

Single-leg lift.

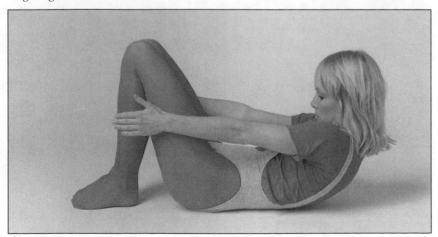

Curl.

Intermediate Level

1. **Hip Roll:** Lie on your back with your arms held out at your shoulders. Bring both your knees in tight to your chest, and slowly roll to your left side with your knees pointed up toward your elbow. Hold your knees 1 to 2 in. off the floor; don't let them touch the floor. Return to the center, roll to your right side, return to the center, and return both your legs to the floor to a full reclining position. Repeat left, center, right, center, floor. Keep your head, shoulders, and upper back on the floor as much as possible.

2. **Bicycle:** Lie on your back, and support yourself up on your elbows. Lift both your legs up off the floor (only 12 to 15 in.) and slowly move your legs in a bicycle pedaling fashion six times. Relax and repeat. Bend your knees slightly as you pedal to keep the action horizontal. Don't arch your lower back. You can place your hands on your hips to help keep your back in contact with the floor.

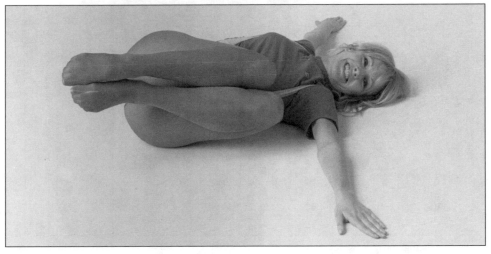

Hip roll.

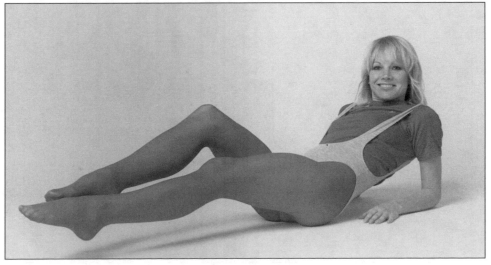

Bicycle.

Advanced Level

1. **Trunk Twisting Sit-Up:** Sit with your knees bent, your feet flat on the floor, and your hands on your shoulders. Turn to your left as far as possible, and slowly curl backward toward the floor (don't touch the floor). Pause, then remain twisted as you slowly curl up to a sitting position. Quickly turn to your right, and repeat the sit-up. Repeat in succession to the left, right.

2. **Seat Walk:** Sit with your knees bent and your arms held out level to your shoulders with your elbows slightly bent for balance. Bring your knees toward your chest and scoot along the floor by lifting and moving from one side of your buttocks to the other. Keep your feet up off the floor. Use your arms and torso to increase your forward motion. Try to seat walk for several feet, then relax and repeat.

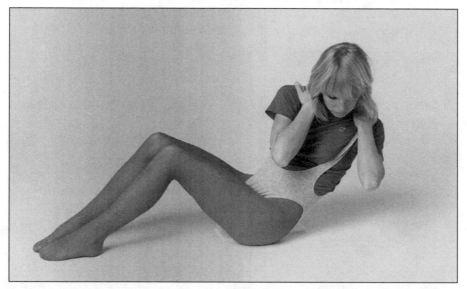

Trunk twisting sit-up.

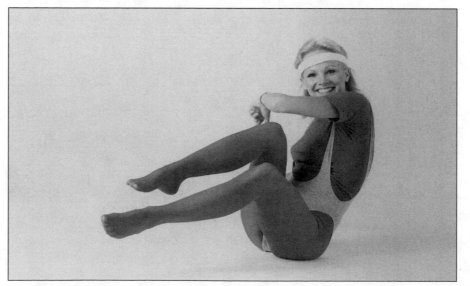

Seat walk.

LEGS

Beginning Level

1. **Side-Lying Single-Leg Lift:** Lie on your left side with legs together and your right hand on the floor in front of you for support. Bend your feet up toward your shins (do not point your toes), and place your right big toe slightly behind your left heel. Slowly lift your right leg up 8 to 10 in. Pause, then slowly lower your leg to the starting position. Repeat in succession, then do the exercise on your other side. Try to lift very slowly and not too high. Also try to keep your body in a straight line on the floor while lifting your legs—do not let your hips roll forward or backward.

2. **Hand-Knee Leg Lift:** Kneel on your hands and knees. Extend your right leg backward along the floor with your toes pointed. Lift your right leg up slowly about 12 to 15 in. (to about hip level). Pause, then slowly lower your leg to touch the floor. Continue lifting and lowering in succession. Repeat the exercise with your left leg. Keep your back straight and your head up throughout the exercise. Kneeling on a padded surface will help cushion your knees.

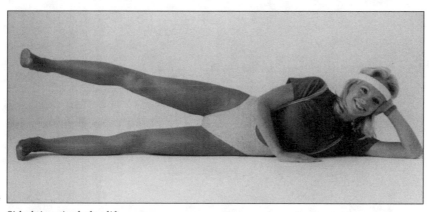

Side-lying single-leg lift.

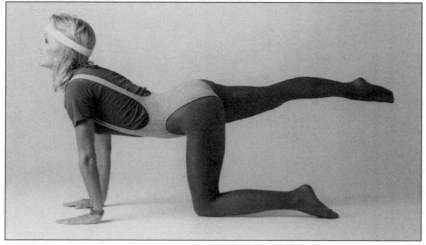

Hand-knee leg lift.

Intermediate Level

1. **Side-Lying Inner-Leg Lift:** Lie on your left side with your left leg extended on the floor and your right leg bent; your right foot is on the floor behind your left knee. Place one hand on the floor in front of you for support. With your left foot bent up toward your shin, slowly lift your left leg up as far as possible. Pause, then slowly lower your left leg back to the starting position. Repeat the exercise with your left leg. Next, repeat the exercise on the other side with your right leg. Keep your body in a straight line on the floor while exercising—don't roll forward or backward.

2. **Doggie Exercise:** Kneel on your hands and knees. Lift your left bent knee up to the side (Position #1), quickly extend your whole left leg straight out to your side as far as possible (Position #2). Return to the bent knee position (Position #3), and back to the starting position (Position #4). Repeat with your right leg, left, right, in succession. Keep your head up, and keep your foot pointed up toward your shin while exercising. Kneeling on a padded surface will help cushion your knees.

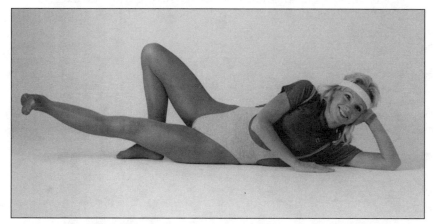

Side-lying inner-leg lift.

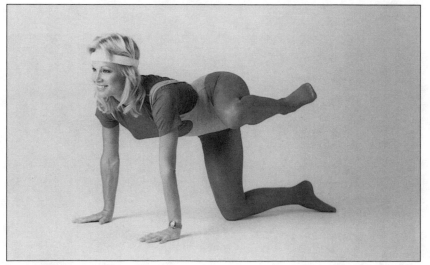

Doggie exercise.

Advanced Level

1. **Flutter Kick:** Lie on your stomach and put your head on your crossed arms in front of you. Point your toes, lift both legs up off the floor and flutter kick for 4 to 6 counts. Return your legs to the starting position, relax, and repeat the kick. Keep your head on your arms, don't bend your knees while kicking, and try not to arch your back. If this exercise bothers your back, do not do it!

2. **Combination Side-Lying Leg Lift:** Lie on your left side with legs together and your right hand on the floor in front of you for support. With your toes pointed up toward your shins, slowly lift your right leg upward 8 to 10 in. and hold. Now, slowly lift your left leg up to touch your right leg, hold, and slowly lower both legs to the starting position. Repeat lifting and lowering your legs in succession. Repeat the exercise on your right side. Be sure to keep your body in a straight line while exercising.

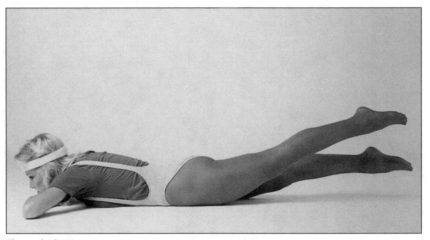

Flutter kick.

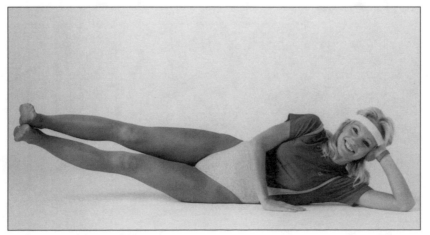

Combination side-lying leg lift.

BUTTOCKS (HIPS)

Beginning Level

1. **Single-Knee Crossover:** Lie on your back with your arms held out at your shoulders. Bend your right knee in close to your chest, and slowly cross it over to your left so that your knee touches the floor. Pause, then slowly lift your knee back to the chest position, and then to the starting position. Repeat with your left knee, right, left, in succession. Try to do this exercise slowly and with control.

2. **Heel Roll:** Lie on your stomach, resting your head on your arms. Your legs are slightly apart and relaxed so that your heels point outward and your toes are touching. Now contract your gluteals by squeezing your buttocks together, rolling your heels inward until they are touching. Hold, relax (your heels will roll outward), and repeat the contraction.

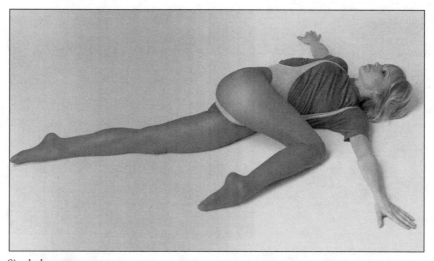

Single-knee crossover.

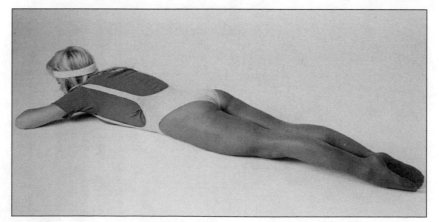

Heel roll.

Intermediate Level

1. **Front-Lying Single-Leg Lift:** Lie on your stomach, resting your head on your hands. Slowly squeeze your buttocks together and lift your left leg 8 to 10 in. up off the floor—keeping your toes pointed. Pause, then slowly lower your leg to the starting position. Relax and repeat lifting with your right leg, left leg, right, in succession. Don't try to lift either leg too high because you may hyperextend (arch) your lower back, which is not only uncomfortable, but places stress on your back.

2. **Single-Leg Crossover:** Lie on your back with your arms held out at your shoulders. Slowly raise your right leg up with your toes pointed, pause, and then lower it across your body toward your left hand. If you can't reach your hand, touch the floor at your waist level. Slowly return your leg to a straight up position and then slowly down to the starting position. Repeat with your left leg, right, left. Keep your head and upper body in contact with the floor during the exercise.

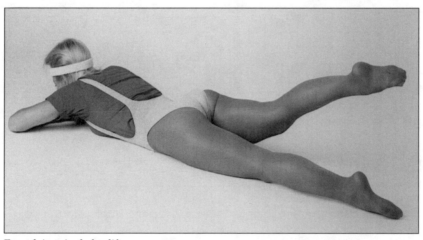

Front-lying single-leg lift.

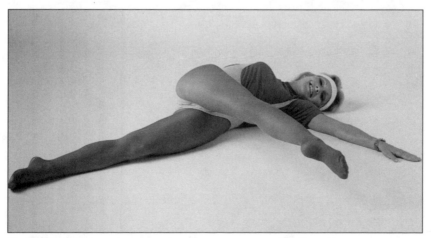

Single-leg crossover.

Advanced Level

1. **Hand-Knee Leg Swing:** Kneel on your hands and knees. Extend your left leg backward along the floor with your toes pointed. Now lift your left leg up, and swing it to your left and back toward your right—behind your supporting right knee. Repeat with the right leg. Keep your head up and back straight while exercising.

2. **Front Support Single-Leg Lift:** Support yourself on your hands and the balls of your feet; slowly lift and lower your right leg, left leg, right, in succession. Keep your toes pointed, your head up, and your back straight. Squeeze your buttocks together while lifting, and don't let your hips and back sag in the middle.

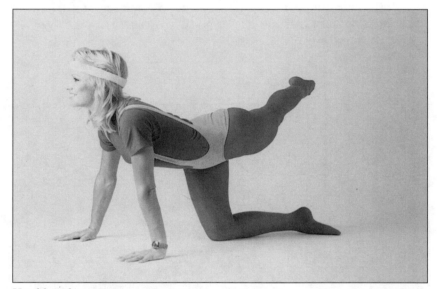

Hand-knee leg swing.

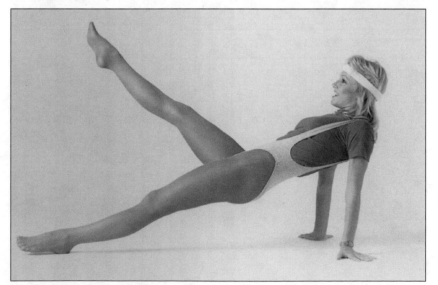

Front support single-leg lift.

ARMS

Beginning Level

1. **Isometric Arm Pull and Push:** Sit or stand comfortably with your arms held out at shoulder level and elbows bent; grasp your fingertips together, and pull one against the other as hard as possible for 4 to 6 seconds. Relax, and shake loose. Then, place the heels of your hands together with fingers extended, and push your palms together hard for 4 to 6 seconds. Relax, and shake loose. Repeat the pull and push in succession. Keep your hands at chest level, and sit or stand straight throughout the exercise.

2. **Wall Push-Up:** Stand about arm's distance from a wall with your hands on the wall at or just above eye level, with your fingertips touching. Keep your heels on the floor and your body straight. Slowly move your body toward the wall with your arms bending until your forehead touches your hands. Push against the wall and extend your arms, moving your body slowly backward to the starting position. Repeat the wall push-ups in succession.

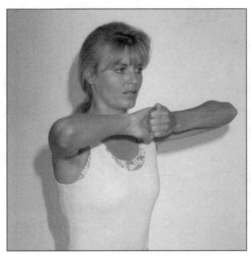

Isometric arm pull (a) and push (b).

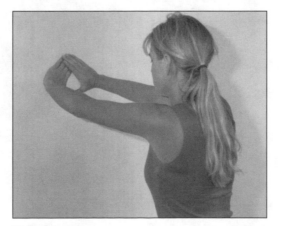

Wall push-up.

Intermediate Level

1. **Standing Arm Circle:** Stand straight with your feet together and arms held out at your shoulders, with your hands in a fist. Slowly make large circles with both your arms forward in succession, and then backward in succession. Relax, and repeat circles forward and backward. Stand tall with your head up throughout the exercise.

2. **Negative-Only Push-Up:** Lean forward on the floor by supporting your body on your extended arms and feet. To begin, slowly lower your chest to the floor using a 3- or 4-second count. Rest momentarily, letting your body touch the floor. Then, as quickly as possible, return to the starting position, *not* by pushing back up with your arms, but by transferring your weight momentarily to your knees and thighs and then reassuming the starting rest position. You are ready to do another negative-only push-up. Repeat in succession. The same arm muscles are used to lower your body as to raise it. The negative or lowering phase of a push-up is considerably easier because you don't have to work against gravity as you do during the positive or pushing upward phase.

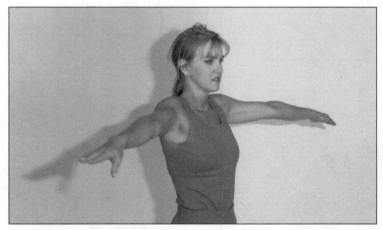

Standing arm circle.

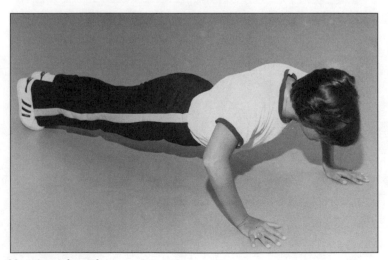

Negative-only push-up.

Advanced Level

1. **Arm Lifting Sequence:** Sit comfortably with your arms down at your sides. With your palms down, slowly lift both your arms out and upward to your shoulder level. Pause, turn your palms up, and continue lifting your arms over your head until your palms are together. Pause, turn your palms out and downward; lower your arms again to shoulder level. Pause, turn your palms up, and lower your arms to the starting position at your sides. Repeat arm lifting in sequence, palms down, palms up, palms together, palms down, palms up. Move slowly and sit straight with your head up and eyes forward. This sequence is designed to help develop arm tone as well as coordination.

2. **Push-Up:** With your body supported on your extended arms and toes, slowly lower your chest to the floor by bending your elbows. Return to the starting position by straightening your elbows. Keep your back straight and your head up; don't let your hips or thighs touch the floor while you are doing push-ups. Repeat in succession, barely touching your chest to the floor with each push-up.

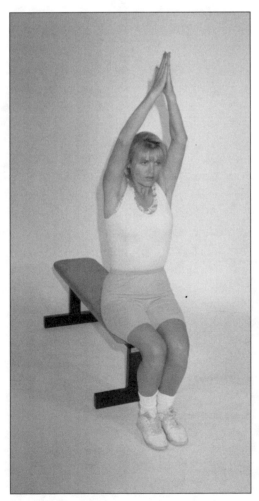

Arm lifting sequence.

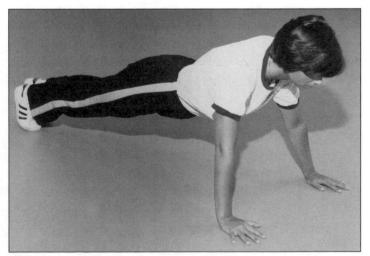

Push-up.